Compulsive Overeating Help

How to Stop Food Cravings, Food Addiction, or Emotional Eating in 6 Simple Steps!

Dennis E. Bradford, Ph.D.

Some Readers' Comments

"Wow!! Finally, someone understands that losing weight is NOT about dieting and deprivation. It's about using your brain and developing new strategies for improving your life. I can honestly say that if you're willing to put the effort in, this really works. The bonus is that these ideas and standards can be applied to many other personal objectives too. Wonderful!!" Mark A. Keicher

"Dr. Bradford received his PhD in philosophy . . . What Dr. Bradford is able to do so very successfully in this books is take an approach which most of us might consider as esoteric (philosophy) and make it pragmatic to our daily lives . . . And Dr. Bradford does it in an easy to read, conversational style, which leads one to silently nod their head in agreement and say to themselves, "yeah, I get it." Central to his premise is that individuals need to believe in themselves to accomplish anything in life; we must have purpose, not just go through the motions. From there, he takes the reader step-by-step, with appropriate exercises, to a path to "killing cravings" (obsessive behaviors . . . Having just read the book, and being someone that has packed "an extra 20 for the past 20", I am anxious to put his methods into practice." Pawel Fludzinski, Ph.D.

"This approach worked well for me and for others to whom I recommended the method. Therefore, I can recommend ths book to anyone who is serious about losing weight and keeping it off. The 6 steps are set out clearly. All that you need to do is to follow the steps. There's a lot of practical wisdom . . . reading it is an excellent way to invest in yourself, your health, and your future." Anna Johnson

"This is a wonderful, thought provoking book! As I started reading, I found myself taking the time to search my soul, reflect, understand and learn on how to improve my overall life. . . [It] not only helps you tackle overeating issues, but has wonderful insight on restoring balance in your life. I found this is a great book to read over again and again. Not only for the reinforcement factor, but found it opened up new ways of positive thinking. I highly recommend this book!" Nancy J.

"Not only does Dr. Bradford explain why we need to liberate ourselves from food craving, but he shows us how to gain the freedom that comes with it. When I first saw this book, I thought "Oh no, not another diet book." But, was I ever wrong. This is a book full of practical solutions to eliminating food cravings, to recognize the thoughts that fail, to create a winner's mind, and to take better control of eating, fitness, R & R, strength, encounters and thoughts. . ." Kathleen T. Dillenbeck

"Overcoming our food cravings, food addictions and emotional eating will help us achieve our ideal weight and prevent us from having life-threatening diseases. This book does not only offers practical advice on how to beat our compulsive overeating habits but shares a lot of insightful information on how to restore the balance in our life that is causing these food cravings and addictions." The Joyful Reviewer

[Reviews from Amazon.com]

Publisher's Notes

This book is for educational, informational, and reference purposes only. The views expressed are those of the author alone, and they should not be taken as expert instruction or commands. This book is intended as entertainment; it contains no professional advice of any kind. Responsibility for any use of the information contained herein is solely the reader's. Although the author and publisher have done their best to provide accurate information, because neither the author nor the publisher has a clue about whether or not you are going to take any action whatsoever based on the powerful information contained in this book or whether it is suitable for you, any liability for damages due to the use of the information contained herein is solely the reader's. The author and publisher make no representation or warranty with respect to the accuracy, applicability, fitness, or completeness of the information in this book. It contains no medical, legal, or accounting advice. The author and publisher shall in no event be held liable for any loss or other damages including, but not limited to, special, incidental, or consequential damages.

Any and all product names referenced within this book are the trademarks of their respective owners. None of those owners has sponsored, authorized, endorsed, or approved of this book. Always read all information provided by the manufacturers' product labels before using any product. The author and publisher are not responsible for claims made by manufacturers.

The author only recommends products that he has personally read or used and found useful. Please do your own due diligence before purchasing anything.

This book is for your own personal use only.

Any perceived slight of any individual or organization is purely unintentional.

This book is a slightly modified second edition of the book entitled "Real Overeating Help" that appeared in 2010.

Printed in the United States of America

Compulsive Overeating Help

How to Stop Food Cravings, Food Addiction, or Emotional Eating in 6 Simple Steps!

"Dig up the root of craving . . ."
The Buddha

"What works, works."
Richard K. Bernstein

Table of Contents

By the Same Author

The Concept of Existence
The Fundamental Ideas
A Thinker's Guide to Living Well
Mastery in 7 Steps
How to Survive College Emotionally
A Dark Time
Personal Transformation
The Three Things the Rest of Us Should Know about Zen Training
The Meditative Approach to Philosophy
How to Eat Less – Easily!
How to Stop Emotional Eating
How to Become Happily Published
Belly Fat Blast with Anna Wright
Getting Things Done
Weight Lifting
Emotional Eating
Love and Respect
12 Publicity Mistakes that Keep Marketers Poor
It's Not Just About the Money!

To

The Ven. Bodhin Kjolhede, Roshi

Acknowledgements

I thank all those students from my courses for over thirty years who struggled to live better, shared with me stories from their lives, and inspired me to try harder to be a more effective teacher and a better human being.

I thank Anna Walker-Wright, Nancy Johncox, Diane J. Keicher, Ky Keicher, Charles A. McLaughlin, Laurie Polito, and Thomas Seem for their comments on earlier versions of the typescript.

Of course, I alone am responsible for any remaining errors.

Preface

Should you read this book?

I don't know.

However, if your enjoyment of life is undermined by having to endure any of the following conditions or diseases, the ideas presented in this book may be very useful to you:

- Food cravings such as cravings for sugar, carbohydrates, or dairy products
- Binging on foods such as sweets
- Obesity
- Hypertension (high blood pressure)
- Type 2 diabetes, pre-diabetes, or genetic susceptibility to diabetes
- Cardiovascular diseases
- Systemic lupus erythematosus or other autoimmune diseases
- Irritable bowel syndrome
- Celiac disease
- Acne
- Allergies
- Menopause symptoms
- Asthma
- Inflammation
- Arthritis
- Joint pains
- Epilepsy
- Mood disorders
- Susceptibility to prolonged bouts of negative emotions such as anger, grief, fear, guilt, sadness, or loneliness
- Lack of cardiovascular fitness

- Lack of physical strength
- Attachment to psychoactive, nonprescription drugs (including alcohol)
- Unstable mood swings
- Bad dreams
- Sleepwalking
- Talking during sleep
- Crying spells
- Blurred vision
- Frequent thirst
- Headaches
- Forgetfulness
- Muscle aches
- Confusion
- Nervous stomach
- Insomnia
- Poor sleep
- Excessive fatigue
- Nervous exhaustion
- Indecision
- Inability to work under pressure
- Depression
- Paranoia
- Dizziness
- Light-headedness
- Anxiety
- Tremors
- Night sweats
- Heart palpitations
- Noticeable lift after one alcoholic drink
- Antisocial feelings such as avoiding social situations or feeling withdrawn around others
- Irritability
- Sudden anger

- Low energy
- Blowing events out of proportion
- Poor memory
- Inability to concentrate
- Sleepiness after meals
- Difficulty awakening in the morning

There are no guarantees. It's impossible to know in advance whether or not a specific behavioral change in a particular individual will reduce or eliminate a certain problem. Nevertheless, learning and adopting the 6 steps presented in this book <u>may</u> alleviate or eliminate any of these difficulties.

Since some of the 6 steps have been used successfully as therapies for all these conditions, it certainly would not be surprising if they helped you.

Furthermore, as long as you have your physician's approval in advance, they almost certainly won't make any of these conditions worse.

If you have any of them, you have the opportunity to understand what has gone wrong and, possibly, cure it and help others who are in distress to do the same.

Even if you are fortunate enough not to have any of them, adopting the 6 steps may prevent you from ever having to endure them. Although we humans are typically much more interested in cures than prevention, that's really a foolish procedure. It's almost always better to prevent a problem from arising than it is to have to deal with it after it has arisen.

If you happen to know someone else who could use some help, I hope that you'll let that person know about this book.

Conesus, New York

1: Freedom from Cravings

Freedom from cravings is your birthright, but you have to claim it.

Why bother to claim it?

Imagine this: you are about to get married and it's moments before the big ceremony. Suddenly you have a strong urge to use a toilet! Cravings undermine the enjoyment of living.

The health consequences alone of not freeing yourself from food cravings are staggering. The unhealthier you are, the more difficult it is to live well. Living well is living freely; being subject to cravings is living poorly.

Food cravings can lead to overeating. Frequent overeating can lead to becoming overweight or obese. Two out of three Americans are overweight or obese.

Although researchers now understand how to prevent type 2 diabetes, 1400 people are diagnosed <u>daily</u> in the United States with diabetes. Diabetes is a symptom of high blood sugar, which is listed as the third leading cause of death in the United States and, because its incidence may be under-reported, it may actually be the leading cause of death.

In addition to negative health conditions like high blood sugar and the other diseases of civilization such as heart attacks, obesity, cardiovascular disease, and strokes, overeating can have important adverse social, financial, and psychological effects. This work is for educational and information purposes only.

Any liability for damages due to the use of the information contained herein is solely the reader's. In other words, you are solely responsible for your own behavior. In particular, it is the reader's responsibility to obtain the blessing of a health care professional before changing any dietary or exercise habits. You are unique. Only your personal physician or other licensed health care professional is in a position to recommend, based on a thorough physical examination, which therapies are advisable for you.

I show you in this book how to free yourself from the food cravings that stimulate emotional overeating in 6 simple steps.

Since you will also learn the principles behind those steps, you will also learn **how to undermine** other kinds of **cravings**.

In fact, I suggest that you don't settle merely for liberating yourself from food cravings. That's a terrific first step, but why not adopt for yourself the goal of liberating yourself from all cravings?

Is anything more important than freedom?

There are 18 specific exercises that will help you turn your improved understanding into real world results. If all you do by reading this book is to improve your understanding, you will have wasted your time. Unless you improve what you do and begin to enjoy concrete benefits, you won't really have learned anything.

So please don't skip any of the exercises. Because you'll need them in the last chapter, save the written exercises.

Since lasting behavioral change is not easy, I devote considerable care in Chapters 2 through 5 to making it as easy as possible for you.

Cravings are intense desires, powerful yearnings. How would you feel if you learned what to do whenever you were assaulted by one? How would you feel if, for the rest of your life, you could diminish the frequency with which they occur or even eliminate them?

Such **peace of mind is priceless.**

Strengthening the ability to focus is the critical step in achieving persistent peace of mind. Since that ability depends upon your brain, the skills involved in improving how you treat and use your brain are the skills required to kill cravings. These skills are of three kinds.

When I was a boy my parents enrolled me in the local YMCA. For years it seemed that I spent every Saturday there. The Y's logo was a three-sided triangle; the sides were labeled "Body," "Mind," and "Spirit."

The kinds of skills required to kill cravings are physical, mental, and spiritual.

Your brain, of course, is part of your body. The **physical** (bodily) skills are those required to have a healthy brain and body. Without having a healthy brain, freedom from cravings is impossible. An unhealthy brain is prone to cravings, addictions, confusion, and other afflictions.

The **mental** (intellectual, conceptual) skills required are those characteristic of having an open mind. Since reality is always in flux, if you are attached to your own static thoughts or even mistake them for reality, your thinking will be delusional. Instead of directly experiencing life, you'll go about locked in a prison of your own thoughts.

The **spiritual** (breathing) skills required are those required for liberation from incessant thinking (conceptualizing). (My use of the word 'spiritual' has nothing necessarily to do with religion and certainly nothing to do with "new age" mumbo jumbo. 'Spiritual' is derived from the Latin 'spititus', which denotes a breath or wind.) If you have ever experienced racing

25

mind insomnia, you have endured attachment to excessive thinking. It is only spiritual skills such as meditation or aliveness awareness that will enable you to liberate yourself from bondage to those emotions that prompt you to use comfort foods to self-medicate.

Since food cravings are desires for physical experiences, it's likely that you are most interested in how to eliminate cravings for physical relief.

Since adults won't normally change what they are doing without understanding *why* they should change as well as *how* to change, reducing cravings for physical relief requires learning why something works. Why would you change if you didn't understand how a proposed change might be beneficial? Understanding such explanations requires mental growth, improving your understanding.

Furthermore, emotional overeating obviously involves emotions. Since they involve both, emotions are neither purely physical nor purely mental. Learning how to deal with those emotions that fuel cravings means learning how to master a breathing practice because breathing is the swinging door between the physical and the mental. Spiritual (breathing) practice will strengthen your ability to focus.

So **the method for killing cravings presented here, "The Killing Cravings Method," necessarily involves the physical, the mental, and the spiritual.**

Therapies that don't involve all three kinds of techniques don't work. They may temporarily provide improvements, but their benefits don't last; they will erode in less than 5 years. They are incomplete. They are too simplistic. They aren't real.

In the United States, the Baby Boomers are the 78 million or so people who were born from 1946 to about 1961 – and there are hundreds of millions of Boomers outside the United States. I myself am a Boomer.

Unlike the generations that follow us, we Baby Boomers should have sufficient life experience not to be taken in by simplistic fad diet or exercise programs that promise much and yield nothing that lasts except disappointment.

Experience by itself is worthless. It's the lessons learned from experience that are valuable. If you fail to learn life's lessons, it will keep trying to teach them to you. You'll stay stuck.

If you are younger than the Baby Boomers, excellent. Reading good books is the fastest way to shorten your learning curve. Why wait to free yourself?

If you are older than the Baby Boomers and willing to learn, it may not be too late to improve the quality of your life – but don't wait to get started until tears are streaming down your cheeks.

If you are sick and tired of being sick and tired, if you are ready to learn the real lessons that experience teaches about how to free yourself from cravings, if you'd prefer liberation from emotions and the cravings they spawn to bondage to them, you are going to treasure this book.

Please set aside your prejudices, attitudes, and beliefs. I don't necessarily imply that they are false; they may not be. Try, though, to separate yourself from them. Please read this whole book with an open mind. **If you aren't willing to improve how you think, you aren't willing to improve the quality of your life.** You have already reached your maximum development. That's unnecessarily sad.

If, *after* reading the whole book, you find that a lot of it makes sense, you are ready to test its ideas for yourself. If it makes little or no sense, pitch it and forget it.

That's fair, isn't it?

Your decisions control the quality of your life, and nobody can make your decisions for you. There's no escape: even if you decide to do what someone else tells you to do, it is you who are deciding to do that.

If you don't improve your decisions now, when will there be a better time to do it?

If you don't follow the experience-based principles presented here, how will you ever do it?

It's good to be skeptical, but, if you are stuck on being negative, you'll just remain stuck. I wholeheartedly encourage you to doubt all the ideas presented here in order to test them for yourself to determine whether or not they'll work for you, too.

They work for me. They have worked for many others. They have been working for a long time. However, you cannot know that they'll work for you until you test them. So, please, be skeptical of the ideas in this book (and, by the way, the ideas promoted by everyone else) and, if they make sense to you, test them for yourself.

Let's begin by ensuring that your thoughts about what to do are serving you well [Chapters 2 through 5]. Then let's examine the physical behaviors that are most effective in killing food cravings [Chapters 6 through 9]. Once you are treating your brain well and beginning to use it better, let's turn to additional practices that yield greater social, emotional, and intellectual stability, which erode from within temptations to overeat [Chapters 10 and 11] before summing up how to get the whole method into action in your life [Chapter 12].

2: Thoughts that Fail

As any good athlete can confirm, if there is anything in your mind except a clear thought that you can complete a difficult task, you'll fail.

I regularly do strength training. Serious strength training involves regularly doing squats, deadlifts, and their variations. Suppose that I am trying a new heavy single deadlift. I have learned many, many times from my own direct experience that, if I do not really believe I can break the bar off the floor and stand up with it, I'll fail to make the lift. Doubt yields failure.

On the other hand, really believing that I can do it does <u>not</u> mean that I'll be able to do it. It is only a necessary, but not a sufficient, condition of doing it.

Similarly, if you improve your understanding about freeing yourself from food cravings or other sorts of cravings, that's not all there is to freeing yourself. You will still need to do whatever it takes.

However, if you fail to improve your understanding about freeing yourself, you will find that you are unable to do it. I don't mean that you will be unable to make any progress. I mean that you will be unable to make any lasting progress.

It's like trying to force a change from the outside instead of letting it grow organically from within.

If you want to try that, be my guest! If your attitude is "just give me the 6 steps," skip ahead to Chapter 6 to learn how to begin implementing the action steps presented in the later chapters of this book.

However, I caution you <u>not</u> to do that. If that's your attitude, please let it go. Believe it or not, adopting the right mindset is more important than the 6 steps.

If you ignore this caution, when your initial success with The Killing Cravings Method begins to reverse itself, please come back here to understand and digest the principles behind the 6 action steps; then, with greater humility, pick yourself up and start again – or give up your dream of freedom and live a diminished life troubled by cravings until you die.

Still here?

Excellent. That's exactly the right way to proceed.

Admit to yourself that your understanding needs to be improved so that you can achieve *lasting* success. After all, you are stuck trying to endure food cravings without giving in to them – and that's very difficult. Nobody thinks that's living well.

Arrogance is common. It requires courage to sustain an open mind.

How many overweight people do you know who say, "I know what to do to lose weight, I just don't do it"? If they really understood how to do it and the consequences of not doing it, they wouldn't be overweight.

If you are arrogant like that, please let it go. If you think you already know it all, you are only obstructing yourself from learning how to improve.

There is so much confused and confusing information being promoted these days that there's no mystery about why you are having problems: you are confused because you are drowning in other peoples' thoughts. Even most well-educated physicians seem clueless when it comes to eating well or improving focus.

Admitting that you need to improve how you think does not mean that all the principles that you have gained from your own experience are false. At least temporarily, however, just set them aside in order to open up to some that may be more effective.

Do you agree to do that? Don't say "yes" with your fingers crossed. Really commit yourself to doing it.

Examining Yourself

Anyone incapable of self-examination or unwilling to do it is incapable of living wisely or well.

To examine yourself is to do your best to admit the truth about yourself. It's being willing to examine all relevant thoughts (judgments, propositions, beliefs, opinions).

Don't worry: you are not your thoughts. You are greater than your thoughts. Since you have the power to change them, you have power over them and are not identical with them.

If you just go along thinking that your thoughts are all true or that your thoughts about reality are themselves reality, you are giving your thoughts power over you. Please don't do that.

It's self-deception. We humans have an unbounded capacity for self-deception, for lying to ourselves. We are wonderful at generating thought after thought even if that means lie after lie.

At least if you want to free yourself from cravings, it's critical to be ruthless in examining your own thoughts. Instead of assuming that they are true, begin examining (testing, probing) them – or, at least, all of them that relate to killing cravings.

Your Self Image

Thoughts that fail to serve you well are all those thoughts that are egocentric, self-centered. These are thoughts you identify with. Why do they fail?

They generate evaluations that are obstructive. (Don't worry: if this isn't already clear to you, it will become much clearer by the end of this book.)

Often, they are thoughts that attempt to limit damage to your self-image. Your "self-image" is your an-

31

swer to the question, "Who am I?" It's the whole set of thoughts that you have about yourself.

Your self-image is made up of dozens and dozens of thoughts about how you are as, for example, a friend, a student, a lover, a parent, a writer, a joke-teller, a driver, a runner, an eater, a walker, a mechanic, a carpenter, and so on.

Why is your self-image important?

I   t's because it's a psychological law that <u>you always behave in accordance with your self-image.</u> Much of what you experience is the result of a self-fulfilling prophecy.

Especially if you have never before encountered that thought, please absorb and digest it.

If you try to effect improvements in your life without first examining and, if necessary, improving your self-image, you will unintentionally sabotage those improvements. By itself, that may explain why some of your past efforts to make lasting improvements have failed.

There is no longer any reasonable doubt that our brains automatically filter and organize our experience. Since what we perceive, remember, and imagine is not as real as we like to believe, what we conceive is frequently dubitable as well.

What's fascinating is that your self-image isn't real. It's just a cluster of thoughts that you have the power to change whenever you decide to change them. Though influential, it's an imaginary picture of yourself, and, because it's imaginary, you can alter it.

Noticing the Automatic

For example, have you walked today the same way you walked yesterday? Since how you walk is a moving autobiographical statement, a close friend could recognize your walk and identify you when you are way off in the distance. After all, you are in the habit of walking the same way every day, aren't you?

Notice that you have the ability to change that whenever you want. Instead of your normal gait, you could walk with the slow, hunched-over walk of someone who is very old, or you could walk with the trained, confident tread of a world-class athlete, or you could stumble along like someone very drunk.

You don't have to walk the way you usually walk. In reality, if you focus on it, you can walk however you choose to walk. Actors do that all the time.

Here's an important point: normally you just walk without thinking about it. Unless you sprain an ankle or injure a leg, you pay no attention to how you walk. You simply walk automatically.

It's not that you cannot be self-conscious of how you walk. You are free to pay attention to it whenever you want to. It's just that, normally, you never do.

In a similar way, **most of what we do is automatic**, most of our behavior is habitual or ritualistic. We don't think about something like walking; we simply do it, and we often do it while thinking about something else.

This is the explanation for much of our boredom and dissatisfaction as well as for our everyday efficiency.

Resetting the Automatic

Lasting improvements are difficult because they involve repeatedly paying attention to what we are doing. If you think that's easy, simply try just holding the same thought in mind for even just a minute or two. (I discuss in Chapter 11 how adopting a certain kind of breathing practice will improve your critical ability to focus, to pay attention, and why that decreases dissatisfaction.)

Lasting improvement requires doing what we don't normally do. It requires temporarily thinking about what we don't normally think about. Whenever we think about it, we are free to change what we are doing. If we repeatedly practice doing something differently, in a few weeks that new behavior will itself become automatic and we won't have to focus so much on it.

Taking Charge

This explains why, if you want to improve the quality of your life, taking charge of your thinking is critical: *your thoughts guide the establishment of your rituals and your rituals, which are what you actually, repeatedly, and automatically do or don't do (including what you think and say), determine the quality of your life.*

This is why it is wise not to skip Chapters 2 through 5 of this book. Anyone who attempts to make lasting behavioral change without first changing thoughts is attempting the impossible. To attempt the impossible is to guarantee failure.

Many thoughtful people have noticed this. Gotama (The Buddha) said, "Our life is shaped by our mind; we become what we think." Ralph Waldo Emerson wrote, "A man becomes what he thinks about most of the time." James Allen wrote, "Act is the blossom of thought . . . " Brian Tracy said, "The quality of your thinking determines the quality of your life."

In fact, even though you may be eager to get to the 6 steps, it's Chapters 2 through 5 that are the most important chapters of this book. Why? Developing the right mindset will enable you to make the best use of the 6 steps. Furthermore, even if I didn't provide them, developing the right mindset would enable you to discover them for yourself. On the other hand, failure to develop the right mindset will undermine their effectiveness.

So, if you want to avoid unintentionally sabotaging your own efforts to free yourself from cravings, first critically examine your thoughts and change them as necessary. That will predispose you to success.

It's not enough just to examine your thoughts. It's necessary to examine them in order to discard those that aren't serving you well.

If this means altering your self-image, alter it.

It can be humiliating to realize that certain thoughts you have had for many years have blocked your progress, but, on the other hand, it is genuinely liberating to let those thoughts go and replace them with better ones.

Your thoughts are not reality. Reality is what it is regardless of your thoughts about it. Your thoughts do not create reality; instead, they create your "surreality," your world, all your personal interpretations of reality.

The truth is that you are inherently free from your thoughts, which means that you are not necessarily bound to them. In practice, this means that, unless you have bound yourself (whether intentionally or not) to your thoughts, what you do or don't do is itself free. Why? You are able to separate yourself from your thoughts in order to control them (while, in turn, they guide your behaviors).

(Of course, your behaviors must be causally possible [and not just logically possible]. For example, if you are paralyzed from the waist down, you will not be able to stand up and walk just by thinking about it.)

Therefore, resolve to take charge of your thoughts. How? Examine them. When you find a thought (or set of thoughts) that isn't serving you well, junk it and replace it with one that may serve you better.

If you stop thinking of your thoughts as true or false, you'll undermine the tendency to think that reality is your thoughts. Think of your thoughts as we have just been doing, namely, as either serving you well or not. <u>Thoughts are replaceable</u>. When you discover that a thought isn't working well for you, replace it.

Nobody (including me) understands your situation better than you do. What is your situation?

Exercise 1

Your first exercise is to examine the following list of thoughts to determine (i) if you believe any of them and, if so, (ii) whether or not they are serving you well.

If, as you do the exercise, these thoughts stimulate other thoughts, examine those other thoughts as well. The idea is to examine the thoughts behind the sentences listed below, which may be the same thoughts behind some of your attitudes.

Be very, very skeptical about believing that any of the following are true. In other words, take seriously the idea of detaching yourself from all these thoughts. Again, they are not you – and simply detaching from them in order to examine them will begin to undermine their power over you.

Here's the list of thoughts to examine. Do you believe any of them – or any others like them?

- I am afraid of living well.
- I am afraid of failing if I really try to live well.
- I am afraid of succeeding if I really try to live well.
- I am not wholly responsible for the quality of my life.
- Because it wins me sympathy from others and is easier, I often think of myself as a victim of circumstances beyond my control.
- I am incapable of killing cravings and, so, incapable of living better.

- I am not pro-active; rather, I am like a leaf in the wind merely reacting to whatever happens.
- I cannot live well because I was too damaged by _____ [fill in the blank with the names of any relevant others such as your parents, teachers, siblings, friends, or lovers].
- I don't have the time to learn how to live better.
- I am lazy and set in my ways, which makes it impossible to live better.
- I have tried to live better before and always failed, so there's no reason to try again.
- I am surrounded by toxic people, so my environment prevents me from living well.
- My self-esteem is too low to live well.
- I am incapable of delaying gratification.
- I am too attached to thinking well to make the effort to put good thinking into action.
- I am irremediably flawed, so there's no point even trying to live better.
- No self-help program works, so there's no reason even to try this one.
- There must be a shortcut to living well, and I'm not going to do anything until I find it.
- The world owes me a good life, and I'm too resentful about the fact that it has so far failed me to do anything to improve myself.
- Nobody else really understands me, so to hell with them and all their ideas about living better.
- Since nothing is perfect, this program to kill cravings isn't perfect -- so there's no point really trying it.
- My way is the best and only way for me.
- I'm smarter than other people, so there's no point in paying attention to them.

- Since having great ideas is easy, living well itself must also be easy and, so, putting in a lot of effort must be counterproductive.
- It's not perfect, but I'm normal and my life is alright just the way it is.

Please sit down by yourself in a quiet place when your mind is fresh and seriously examine those beliefs that actually constitute your attitudes. Try to figure out if any have been obstructing you.

Do you understand that all the thoughts listed, and many other similar ones, are nothing but supposedly self-serving excuses?

None of them are genuinely self-serving. Attaching yourself to any will undermine your attempt to free yourself from cravings even before you begin.

Plato was the first great philosopher in the western tradition. (A philosopher is a lover of wisdom, in other words, someone who seriously wants to live well.) "[T]he life of a philosopher," Socrates says in Plato's *Apology* is "to examine myself and others."[1]

No examination, no wisdom; no wisdom, no living well.

Socrates, Plato's teacher, believed that the really important thing is not to live, but to live well.

Living wisely or well requires detaching from your own thoughts in order to examine them. It requires escaping from the tyranny of your own thoughts, especially from those thoughts that obstruct living freely, which includes cravings.

Freedom is not free. Freeing yourself from bondage to your thoughts begins by distancing yourself from them, examining them, letting go of those that aren't serving you well, and replacing them with ones that may serve you well. Test the new ones and, if they also fail, replace them and continue the process. This is living an examined life.

Freedom requires living an examined life.

The only alternative to the examined life is the unexamined life. **Living an examined life is a necessary, but not a sufficient, condition of living well.** Living an unexamined life is a sufficient condition of failing to live wisely or well.

As Socrates says in Plato's Apology, "to let no day pass without discussing goodness and all the other subjects about which you hear me talking and examining both myself and others is really the very best thing that a man can do, and . . . life without this sort of examination is not worth living."[2]

If we want to live wisely or well, living an examined life is not just our duty to ourselves. In Plato's *GORGIAS* Socrates tells us that it is also our duty to our fellows: speaking of "persuading and coercing fellow citizens to the point of self-improvement," he says, "this and this alone is the task of a truly good citizen."[3]

So, at least if you would follow Socrates and other philosophers, resolve to examine yourself, your thoughts and your behaviors, every day and to help others do the same.

Becoming wise begins with self-examination.

There's no other way to wisdom.

Getting Even More From This Book

As you encounter new ideas, notice any emotional reaction you have to them.

Does a new idea threaten or frighten you? Does it anger you? Do you immediately want to blame whoever suggested it? Does it excite you? Do you immediately want to share it with a loved one?

Our emotions are more important than we often like to think. We pretend that our rationality controls our emotions when it is usually the other way round.

So noticing your own emotional reactions to the ideas presented here is a way of learning about yourself.

If you will do that, you will not just learn about curbing overeating, you will learn more about other automatic behaviors that may not be serving you well.

In this way, reading this book can also be an important way to examine yourself.

3: A Winner's Mind

You are already a winner. If you don't think so, the problem is only that you don't yet realize it.

You may not realize it because your own thoughts are obscuring your insight. You may be so confused that, instead of directly experiencing life, you often live in your own thoughts, or, to put it differently, you often live in your own head or mind.

If so, it's normally as if your thoughts and your behaviors are separated.

Separation is the cause of dissatisfaction (discontent, suffering, unhappiness). The less separation you experience, the less dissatisfaction you'll need to endure.

The good news is that life is much more enjoyable than you may think it is.

To use an example from the last chapter, when you walk you are usually behaving in a certain way without really thinking about what you are doing. If you are walking to work or to the laundry room or inside a store, you may be thinking about what might occur at work or your next laundry chore or wondering where in the store the item is that you came in to buy.

What's wrong with that?

Let me encourage you to discover the answer to that question for yourself. Here's the exercise.

Exercise 2

Cast your thoughts back over your life until you find some well-rehearsed behaviors in which you just *were* the behavior. These are sometimes called "*optimal experiences.*"

In an optimal experience, there is no gap between your thinking and your doing. Since there's no separation, there's no dissatisfaction. It's a taste of what life as a sage is like. (A "sage" is a successful philosopher, in other words, someone who is wise and lives well.) You are wholly absorbed in the activity. Instead of being self-conscious about what you are doing, you *are* the activity.

I   n an optimal experience, life flows. It seems spontaneous and feels joyful. Consciousness of the passing of time evaporates. There's no need for trying because you are already fully absorbed in the experience. Instead of being scattered, your mind is unified.

The key to recalling optimal experiences is to look for only well-rehearsed behaviors. Such behaviors are the result of specific training that you deliberately repeated over and over again.

Did you ever learn how to play a musical instrument? You cannot think your way to playing it well; you must practice it. To become good, you must practice playing it daily, or nearly daily, for a long time. Furthermore, you must practice properly, and you must practice for a sufficient length of time. (Typically, daily sessions will last no less than thirty minutes and the first optimal experience may not occur for years.) If, as a child, you spent some years, say, practicing the piano or the violin daily and you eventually became so good that you really enjoyed it, there were probably times when "it" happened.

Although "it" seems to happen spontaneously and it is impossible to predict when it will happen, it's always the result of well-rehearsed behaviors. It's **the shift from trying** to play the instrument **to being** the playing of the instrument.

The same thing occurs when learning a skill for a sport. My game was hockey. As a boy, I tried to develop a quick, hard, accurate wrist shot. I practiced it over and over and over for many hockey seasons. Eventually, there were times during a game when my ego/I disappeared into the shooting of the puck. At least occasionally, "I" would simply make the right shot automatically. Instead of trying to make the shot, I just did it. I was the shooting.

"It" is being in that kind of zone.

If you have never experienced it, your education was deficient.[4] If you have experienced it, you don't need me to attempt to describe it further.

Back to walking.

Exercise 3

Try this: take off any shoes or socks that you happen to be wearing and go for a walk barefoot for a few minutes. Forget about everything else except walking. Focus only on your walking. Walk slowly.

Notice the sensations as one foot lands on its heel and your weight is transferred forward to the next step. Notice how the carpet, the tile, the wood or the earth feels as you tread on it—and how those feelings change when the surface you are walking on changes. Notice how you breathe as you walk, and how you naturally move your arms. Really, for perhaps the first time as an adult, try to enjoy the direct experience of walking. Imagine what it would be like never to enjoy walking again.

Don't just think about this exercise. If you actually do each of the exercises as they arise in order in this book, you'll benefit much more than just from reading it. I really want you to succeed and not just think about succeeding.

Question: did you enjoy your walking more when you were paying attention to it (as opposed to being lost elsewhere in thought)?

Similarly, do you enjoy eating a peach more when you are paying attention to what you are doing or when you are thinking about something else? What about drinking a soda, having sex, feeling a cool breeze on your face on a hot day, or taking a bath?

The key to wisdom is paying full attention to the present moment. Doing that ends separation and, so, dissatisfaction.

Distinguish 'pain' from 'suffering.' I use 'pain' to refer to physical pains like being hungry, having a headache, enduring a fever, or breaking a bone. Pain happens; it's an inevitable part of life. Suffering, though, is optional [see Chapter 11].

Here's the principle: sometimes what you are <u>not</u> doing is more important for success than what you <u>are</u> doing. If you simply let your thoughts run on and on so they go wherever they will, then that failure to discipline them, that failure to pay attention to what is actually happening, by itself, is sufficient to explain your lack of success so far in a specific domain.

Mihaly Csikszentmihalyi: "To control attention means to control experience, and therefore the quality of life."

How?

When you are in doubt about a perplexing matter, like all philosophers Gotama (The Buddha) recommends that you should examine a way of life for yourself by paying greater attention to your own experience. For example, he famously recommended: "Do not go by oral tradition, by lineage of teaching, by hearsay, by a collection of texts, by logic, by inferential reasoning, by reasoned cogitation, by the acceptance of a view after pondering it, by the seeming competence of a speaker, or because you think, 'The ascetic is our teacher.' But when you know for yourselves, 'These things are unwholesome; these things are blamable; these things are censured by the wise; these things, if undertaken and practiced, lead to harm and suffering,' then you should abandon them."5

The future need not resemble the past. Failing to succeed yesterday does not entail failing to succeed today or tomorrow.

Evaluations, which are judgments about good and bad, are nothing but thoughts. Unless you attach to them, they are never obstacles. However, if you attach to them, they can be major obstacles.

If you attach to the thought "I am a failure," you will always tend to act in accordance with that belief. It works the same way for the thought "I am a success."

The best procedure for living wisely or well is regularly detaching from your thoughts in order to enjoy direct experience. If, instead, you choose to be bound by your thoughts, you are, presumably without realizing it, putting yourself in bondage. It's impossible to live freely while living in bondage.

The second best procedure for living wisely or well is to examine your thoughts in order to discipline them to ensure that they are always serving you well.

At least as an adult, unless you give it to them, nobody else has any power whatsoever over your thoughts.

When it comes to problem solving, your thoughts are invaluable. However, it's counterproductive to attach to them. **Wisdom requires using instrumental reason without overusing it. So it requires a middle way.**

It makes no difference that your parents and early environment weren't perfect, that attachment to some of your so-called friends has been holding you back, that your teachers and professors were less than ideal, and so on. Life has dealt you a unique set of assets and liabilities. Your task is to discover them through self-examination and make the most of what you've been given.

Commit yourself wholeheartedly: "if it is to be, it's up to me." Please forget about blaming either others or yourself. Again, negative evaluations are just thoughts. Decide that your specific circumstances and other externals don't count. Suck it up and assume full responsibility from now on for the quality of your life.

Have you so far failed to work hard enough? If so, don't get stuck there; instead, get started. Work hard and persistently to give a method (technique, procedure, program) a good shot. What if it still doesn't work?

Failure is nothing but negative feedback. All it means is that what you have been doing so far hasn't worked. It doesn't mean that there's something inherently wrong with you (there isn't) and it doesn't mean that something else won't work. So adjust what you are doing in accordance with the feedback you've been getting and work hard and persistently in a different way.

For example, if your percentage of body fat is too high, adjust what you are doing to discover how to get a better result. It's not a matter of theory; it's a matter of what works. Whatever works, works.

How do you feel about yourself? Overeating can be a means of coping with low self-esteem. If you happen to have low self-esteem, realize that you weren't born that way. Your learning to have bad feelings about yourself was not your fault. The good news about self-esteem is that it is possible to increase it permanently. It's an important obstacle that you should remove.[6]

Becoming More Skillful

A sage is simply someone who is wise, someone who has mastered a certain skill set. Becoming wiser, living better, is only a matter of learning better skills.

Have you ever tried hard to develop a skill when you lacked the talent for it? If you don't have a head for mathematics and tried to major in it at college, by the time you reached third semester calculus you started looking for another major If you are no good at hitting a curve ball and tried to become a position player in professional baseball, you soon went looking for employment elsewhere.

We all have different abilities and disabilities.

The lesson is <u>discover your aptittudes and develop them into skills</u>.

How could your life flow if you are always struggling to turn weaknesses into skills?

If you are not sure what your talents are, here are three ways to uncover them.

First, and this is the most important one, think back to your school days. The purpose of education is to discover aptitudes and develop them into skills. What came more easily to you than it did to others? What were you naturally good at doing? Your answer will provide important clues.

Second, ask people who know you well. Ask your parents, siblings, and long time friends what your best talents are. Once you convince them that you are not going to take their answers personally, they'll tell you. Don't argue with their answers or get defensive; instead, genuinely thank them and then seriously consider their replies.

Third, take aptitude tests and read relevant books. If you are willing to do a bit of research and spend a little money, it's now possible to find and take good tests online.[7] There are, of course, plenty of books that will help you examine yourself.[8] Once you are clear about your aptitudes, decide, if you haven't already, which one to develop first into a skill and then work hard to do just that. Master it. How could you feel good about your life if you are not excellent at something?

"Hard work" does not mean "incessantly hard work." Hard work should always be balanced with focused recovery and renewal. If you always seem to be working hard and yet always are struggling, perhaps what you have identified as an aptitude isn't really an aptitude.

By "hard work" I do, though, mean regularly focusing on improving your skill. If you are not practicing a new skill for an hour or two daily, how serious are you about mastering it?

Don't worry: I suggest important new skills later in this book that are necessary for everyone who wants freedom from cravings. The most important new skill is described last [in Chapter 11]. With respect it, you already have the necessary aptitude and there's no need for you to re-invent the wheel, in other words, there's no need for you to develop a new technique to turn that aptitude into a skill. The method for transforming that critical aptitude into a skill has been available for millennia.

The good news here is that, once you master it, what used to be hard work will seem like play. That's a key sign of mastery.[9]

Exercise 4

Here are 5 common ways we sabotage ourselves. Do any of them apply to you? Do any relate to your overeating? If so, what action steps might work well for you to stop sabotaging yourself?

This is another exercise in self-examination. Please don't set it aside until later. Because life is short and it's easy to get distracted, *speed of implementation* is a common characteristic of successful people. When they encounter what may be a helpful technique, they immediately apply it, note the feedback they get from applying it, and, when necessary, adjust what they are doing.

Ask yourself these 5 questions and seriously think about their answers. If those answers are not what you'd like them to be, immediately implement steps to cure what you now realize is ailing you.

Do I often get stuck on my own thoughts?

Do I tend to take things personally?

Have I developed a detached attitude?

Do I often fail to acknowledge complexity?

Am I usually reactive rather than proactive?

Let's briefly consider the answers to each of these questions in turn. They are important and may be counter-intuitive to you.

First, if you are frequently getting stuck or fixated on your own thoughts or, even worse, if you frequently mistake them for reality, the way to begin to get unstuck is to *develop the habit of examining your own thoughts.*

Perhaps the most enjoyable way to do that is by discussing them with a wise friend. Since wise friends are few and far between, the most commonly recommended antidote is daily reading in a good book (such as the ones listed in the Selected Bibliography of this book). The idea is to notice persistent thoughts that are afflicting you and to challenge them.

There's reading, and then there's reading. The way to read is to do your best to understand the author's point of view and then, if the author's point of view differs from yours, ask yourself how the author might attack your point of view and what your best reply should be to that criticism. (Don't ever confuse an attack on a view with a personal attack.) In other words, don't read merely to adopt another's point of view. That's not serious reading. Read as if the author were in a conversation with you, as if the author's ideas and your ideas were in combat.

Descartes: "I have been nourished on letters since my childhood . . . I was aware that the reading of all good books is indeed like a conversation with the noblest men of past centuries who were the authors of them, nay a carefully studied conversation, in which they reveal to us none but the best of their thoughts."[10]

Intellectual progress occurs only when ideas clash.

So, if you regularly clash the ideas of supposedly expert authors against your own ideas and think carefully about the results, you are using reading to improve your own thinking. That's how to make friends with great authors. That's how to read.

That advice, of course, also applies to how you should read this book. If my ideas stand up to your initial examination, test them in practice. If they don't actually work well for you, pitch them – and enjoy the greater confidence that comes from having had your ideas stand up to the test of being seriously challenged. If they work well, adopt them.

Never be satisfied with the quality of your own understanding. Assuming you don't have a wise friend to talk with daily, read seriously every day for at least 20 or 30 minutes. 'Every day' means 'until your dotage.' If you don't take advantage of your skill at reading, you might as well be illiterate.

Meister Eckhardt: "There is no stopping place in this life, -- no, nor was there ever for any man no matter how far along his way he'd gone." Sir John M. Templeton: "Only one thing is more important than learning from experience, and that is not learning from experience." Walt Disney: "There is more treasure in books than in all the pirate's loot on Treasure Island . . .and best of all, you can enjoy these riches every day of your life. Warren Buffett: "It has been helpful to me to have tens of thousands turned out of business schools taught that it didn't do any good to think." Roger von Oech: "The best way to get a good idea is to get a lot of ideas."

Second, sages never take things personally. A "sage" is someone who is wise (a successful philosopher, someone who lives well). [I discuss sages more in Chapter 11.] If you are not yet a sage, you will, at least occasionally, be tempted to take things personally.

Don't.

Nothing is personal.

Problems occur. So? Fix them without blaming anyone or anything.

If you have an entitlement mentality, let it go. The world is already open to you; it owes you nothing.

Being egocentric is being immature. Think of children. The cure for egocentricity is mastering any traditional spiritual practice. [I explain in Chapter 11 how to begin to do that.]

The egocentric are takers, whereas selfless sages are givers. Living well is not about gaining anything; *living well is about giving everything.*

Lao-tzu: "The sage does not take to hoarding. / The more he lives for others, the fuller is his life. / The more he gives the more he abounds . . . Is it not because he is selfless / That his self is realized?" Don Miguel Ruiz: "Whatever happens . . . don't take it personally. . . Personal importance, or taking things personally, is the maximum expression of selfishness, because we make the assumption that everything is about 'me.'"

Third, until you develop a detached attitude, you will never live well. There's no such thing as a sage who is not detached. To be attached is to be unbalanced, off-centered. **The more detached you are, the better you'll live.**

Especially if you think of normal emotional attachments formed with family members, this may strike you as counter-intuitive.

Detachment relates to never taking things personally. The critical aspect of being detached is being free from being stuck on yourself, from being attached to your own ego and your own egocentric preferences.

When you free yourself from being attached to incessantly thinking about yourself, you become free to think about others. When you begin focusing on helping others, they'll notice, and your life will improve. [There's more about this in Chapter 10.]

The less you are attached to your own preferences, the more you'll be open to loving other people. Since it is people with low self-esteem who are stuck on themselves, this kind of detachment requires high self-esteem.

This explains why sages, who have achieved the greatest detachment, are also the greatest lovers. To LOVE is to promote what is good for your beloved; it is not to use your beloved to promote what is good for you. To love well is to promote what really is good for your beloved with no expectation of gaining anything in return. Only sages are fully able to love well.

Egocentric evaluative thoughts (such as "this is good for me" or "this is bad for me") are nothing but thoughts. Since they obstruct freedom and love, the wise detach from them.

To develop a detached attitude, begin thinking that everything is a test, that every experience is an experiment. Experiences have consequences that are nothing but grist for your mill, in other words, they are only more feedback. Adjust what you are doing in light of the feedback and proceed.

From The Bhagavad Gita: "Seek refuge in the attitude of detachment." Sengcan: "If you're attached to anything, / you surely will go far astray." Meister Eckhart: "I praise detachment above all love . . . above all humility . . . above all mercifulness." Andrew Matthews: "The challenge of life is to appreciate everything and attach yourself to nothing."

Fourth, life presents us with complicated situations and *always insisting on simplistic answers is the mark of a fool.*

Intelligence is very helpful, but it is over-rated. Being intelligent is not necessary for being wise. You are as intelligent as you need to be.

Getting stuck on simplistic answers, which seems to happen most loudly in the political arena, is just another way of being attached to your own thoughts and egocentric evaluations. Sages are not attached to anything. They certainly don't get stuck in prisons of their own thoughts.

Winston Churchill: "Remember the story of the Spanish prisoner. For many years he was confined in a dungeon . . . One day it occurred to him to push the door of his cell. It was open; and it had never been locked." H. L. Mencken: "For every complex problem there is an easy answer, and it is wrong." Ronald E. Osborn: "Undertake something that is difficult; it will do you good. Unless you try to do something beyond what you have already mastered, you will never grow."

Fifth, if you are incessantly reactive instead of proactive, you have not prioritized what you are doing. You are not clear on which values you hold most dear.

Furthermore, it's a sign that you have never systematically related your ideas. If your life is constantly chaotic, that's the problem. The solution is to **prioritize your values**.

Richard Bandler and John Grinder: "most people are very chaotically organized on the inside." Brian Tracy: "If you don't set goals for yourself, you are doomed to work to achieve the goals of others." Price Pritchett: "Where's the logic in not trying [to fulfill your goals] because you might not succeed, when in not trying you guarantee failure?"

You will genuinely begin to feel like a winner only when you make significant progress towards your goals. So the logically first question to ask yourself is, "What do I want?"

If you don't know where you are trying to go, how will you plan your journey? If you don't plan your journey, how will it take you where you want to go?

Aristotle was Plato's student and the second great philosopher in the western tradition. He pointed out that instrumental reason, which is our chief tool for figuring out how to get what we want, can only work when it is provided with an end (purpose. direction, value) and that it itself cannot provide that end. He argues that there must be "some end of the things we pursue in our actions which we wish for because of itself" (or the justifications for our choices would go on indefinitely – and, so, prove to be no justification at all) and that deciding what this ultimate value is is "also of great importance for the conduct of our lives" because "if, like archers, we have a target to aim at, we are more likely to hit the right mark."[11]

It's important to distinguish "goals" from "Projects."

Goals are concrete events or outcomes that may be achievable such as making a million dollars, bench pressing 300 lbs., or having sex with someone. Instrumental reason is critical in figuring out how to achieve goals.

Projects are ends or general directions in life (ultimate values) that are never finished such as being a parent or being an artist or being loving. Instrumental reason is useless in selecting ends.

To think through your values is to chose your Projects and rank them in order of priority. Once you have done that, select goals in accordance with your Projects.

Cynthia Kersey: "William Marsten, a prominent psychologist, asked 3,000 people, 'What have you to live for?' The results revealed that 94 percent responded by saying they had no definite purpose for their lives – 94 percent! It has been said that 'everyone dies, but not everyone really lives.' Marsten's survey sadly supports that statement." Helen Keller: "Many persons have the wrong idea about what constitutes true happiness. It is not gained through self-gratification but through fidelity to a worthy purpose." Richard Carlson: "Imagining yourself at your own funeral allows you to look back at your life while you still have the chance to make some important changes."

Freedom is a Project. The word 'freedom' is so vague that it is nearly useless without further specifying it. It really involves both positive ends (what freedom is for) as well as negative ends (what freedom is from).

Assuming that you want **freedom from cravings**, The Killing Cravings Method can be part of your Project. Once you choose it, its 6 steps are the result of using instrumental reason to help you attain that goal.

Once you select where you are trying to go, if you focus clearly on your destination, your brain will automatically help you plan your route. It's quite marvelous that way.

You are unique. Your body/mind is unique. The important implication here is that, even if the goal is the same, you may or may not be able to use the same route that worked for someone else.

That's not a problem if you understand that the 6 steps presented in this book are nothing but suggested experiments for you to test. If a step works, keep using it; if one fails, try something else instead.

Confucius: "Our greatest glory is not in never failing, but in rising every time we fail." Samuel Beckett: "No matter. Try again. Fail again. Fail better." Eric Hoffer: "man is most uniquely human when he turns obstacles into opportunities." Price Prtichett: "Usually success is a direct byproduct of screw-ups."

There's no way for you to know in advance which tactics will work best for you to achieve your goals. (I explain why in the next chapter.) Living an examined life means regularly figuring out what is working for you and doing it while letting go of what isn't working for you.

The goal is your target. You will soon have multiple arrows in your quiver to choose to shoot at the goal. If you miss with one arrow, shoot another. So, first, what's your target?

Exercise 5

Write down on paper what you want to achieve in one sentence. Put your goal in positive terms rather than in negative ones.

For example, don't write, "I do not want to have any more food cravings"; instead, write "I want freedom from food cravings." Similarly, instead of writing, "I want to lose 40 pounds," write something like "I want to achieve the body composition I had when I graduated from high school" or "I want to achieve 15% body fat."

Then sit down and brainstorm at least 20 ways that might work for you to achieve and maintain your goal. For now, just write them down without being critical of them, and don't stop until you have at least 20. The last 5 or so may be difficult to come up with, but stick to it until you have at least 20.

John C. Maxwell: "People don't like to admit that they need to change. And if they are willing to alter things about themselves, they usually focus on cosmetic changes." Denis Waitley: "Your imagination is your preview of life's coming attractions."

In order to let your brain work on it, I suggest visualizing success and sleeping on it before you do your brainstorming session.

To visualize is to imagine seeing. It's preferable not to limit yourself to seeing. The idea is to program your brain for success by using all your senses (not just vision) to imagine yourself as the winner you want to be.

This is possible and helpful because your brain cannot distinguish the real from the unreal. Put another way, it cannot distinguish between a positive thought and a negative thought. This is why it is important not to write your goal as a negative thought. If, for example, you write "I do not want to have cravings" and repeatedly focus on that thought, because your brain cannot register the negative you'll actually be training your brain to focus on the thought "I do want to have cravings"!

Several times daily take a few moments, using as much sensory detail as possible, to imagine yourself positively as having already hit your target.

How will you feel? How will your health improve? How much better will you look? Think how pleased you'll be when your physician is astounded at your positive transformation. Think of the compliments from others you'll receive, too. Think how much more energy you'll have. Think how much more easily you'll climb stairs or fit into an airplane seat or dance or even run.

Then pick an option from your list of (at least) 20 and test it. If it begins to work, master it. If it doesn't, pick another option.

This is an exercise in optimism, which may be difficult for you if you are in the habit of habitually adopting a negative attitude. (Pessimistic people usually don't think of themselves as pessimistic; instead, they think of themselves as realistic.) It may even strike you as so much baloney.

Why does this work?

When it comes to public, measurable, or external goals, the more in control we feel, the happier we feel. The less in control we feel, the worse we feel. Investigate them for yourself by recalling specific incidents from your own life when you felt out of control and compare them to times when you felt fully in control.

On the other hand, it's important to note that, when we try to control private or internal goals, we actually make ourselves less happy. In particular, suppressing thoughts backfires. Deliberately trying to control our thoughts creates dissatisfaction.

What works with respect to thoughts is accepting them all, which diminishes their power, and then evaluating them in terms of how well they are working or serving us. It's important not to take them at face value, in other words, not to think of them as truths. Learning how to detach or disentangle yourself from your thoughts is a critical skill required for a significant increase in wisdom. In effect, it involves learning how to avoid a natural misuse of your mind.[12]

To reduce separation is to reduce dissatisfaction. To suppress thoughts is to try to separate from them, which only increases dissatisfaction.

Back to visualizing: Visualize in as much sensory detail as possible how a typical day will go *after* your have hit your target. Imagine being healthier, feeling better, looking better, and tackling your work with more energy and enthusiasm. Imagine, too, how much more attractive you'll be to others.

There is an important tactic, though, for making visualization work: when a negative thought or image pops into your mind, *immediately* replace it with a positive one. Do not get entangled in it by trying to fight it or argue against it; instead, the instant you notice it, drop it and replace it with a positive thought or image.

In fact, this is one of the most important habits you can ever develop. [It's great training for the practice that is discussed in Chapter 11.]
It's impossible to control what life throws at you, but it's possible and desirable to control your reactions to what life throws at you.

To develop a positive attitude, use this deliberate, disciplined way of reacting. This is not the foolish optimism of Voltaire's Candide. This is, to use Price Pritchett's terms, the "hard optimism" of *non-negative thinking*.

You may think that accepting all your thoughts and then evaluating them only on how well they serve you doesn't work. Many people do. The advantage of that kind of negative thinking is that you don't have to bother to discipline yourself. The huge disadvantage of that kind of laziness is that you will perpetually prevent yourself from using the most important arrow in your quiver. Instead of adopting an important mental skill, you fruitlessly keep trying to suppress thoughts that you don't like and continue to be dissatisfied.

Self-talk is just thinking silently to ourselves. Plato wrote in his dialogue Sophist that thinking "is, precisely, the inward dialogue carried on by the mind with itself . . . without spoken word."[13] We all do it frequently, sometimes almost incessantly.

It's how we do it that is extremely important. If you do it by avoiding non-negative thinking, you may amaze yourself at the beneficial outcomes.

Gotama said, "With our thoughts we make the world." (In other words, your thinking creates the world you live in.) The Bible inspired the aphorism: "As a man thinketh in his heart so is he." (In other words, what you say to yourself creates your character.) James Allen: "Suffering is always the effect of wrong thought." Norman Vincent Peale: "Change your thoughts and you change your world." (In other words, you change your surreality -- not reality itself.)

We become what we frequently think to ourselves.

Perhaps the best example of this is self-esteem. Do you like yourself? Do you feel good about being you? Do you love yourself? If so, you have high self-esteem; if not, you have low self-esteem. It's important to have high self-esteem.[14]

If you have low self-esteem, you probably think thoughts like: "If only I had better genes I could kill my food cravings" or "Everything I eat just becomes body fat" or "Whenever I make a plan to reach a goal I never stick to the plan."

If you have high self-esteem, you probably think thoughts like: "I always exercise when it's time to exercise" or "I am in full control of my values and rituals" or "I enjoy setting goals, making plans, and then following those plans to achieve my goals."

If you are familiar with and use positive self-talk, you have already cultivated a very important asset.

If you are unfamiliar with it and would like to learn about it, I recommend Shad Helmstetter's <u>What to Say When You Talk To Yourself</u>. He writes, "Self-Talk is a way to override our past negative programming by erasing or replacing it with conscious, positive new directions."

I suggest using self-talk throughout the day and always using non-negative thinking.

On the other hand, because it is bound by language, self-talk by itself cannot yield peace of mind. So, though it's a valuable tactic, it's value is limited.

Use moderation here, because always trying to obtain goals such as doing better at self-talk is an oppressive way of living.

There are similar techniques worth considering. For example, there is the time-line technique developed in Neuro-Linguistic Programming [NLP]. It's really an extension of goal-setting and visualization that can help bring about a congruency between imagining yourself at a future time and how you think of yourself now. It's easy to find books and audio programs on NLP or even to hire an NLP therapist.

Let me emphasize your uniqueness. Your genetic code is unique. How your brain developed is unique. The experiences you've had in life are unique.

Therefore, don't assume that any specific technique that worked for someone else to achieve the goal that you also want to achieve will work for you. It may or may not. The only way to find out is to test it. If it works for you, terri-fic. If it doesn't, try something else.

It's very important that you not think of yourself as a loser if some technique doesn't work well for you. That would be foolish. Its failure to work well for you is nothing but feedback. Don't take it personally. Just shrug your shoulders and try a different technique. The reality is that you are one step closer to finding a technique that will work for you, so, in that sense, your failure was nothing but an instance of successful learning.

Adopt a probing, testing, curious, experimental attitude. It's the attitude of a philosopher.[15]

The only failure occurs when you quit trying. A lack of persistence is your fault, which means that you can correct it and resurrect hope whenever you decide to.

Please be alert, too, for all-or-nothing thinking. It almost never happens that a method is either a total success or a total failure. This psychological trap of perfectionism snares many people.

For example, if your goal is to eliminate food cravings and you reach the point where you are averaging one food craving monthly, are you a failure? Hardly! That may not be total success, but it is likely to be immensely better than what you are experiencing now. If you are suffering from multiple food cravings daily and are confused about how to handle them, it would be a genuine victory if you could kill most of them and learn how to deal effectively with the occasional one that still occurs.

Set realistic goals. Having one food craving monthly is a more realistic goal than never again ever experiencing a food craving.

In fact, you may already understand how to handle an occasional one when it occurs. Instead of thinking, "I'm such a loser I cannot even eat a piece of cake," immediately replace that thought with something like, "Good. That's a reminder of how far I've come, and I'm glad to be reminded every few weeks of my progress. Thank you, Mind."

Because you don't know what you are doing (I explain why in the next chapter) and big missteps can have disastrous consequences, it's best to make progress in small steps, one at a time. Little successes eventually add up to big successes. As you are taking the small steps, savor each one by noticing how far you've come. Teach yourself how to enjoy the process, and give yourself little rewards along the way to celebrate improvements in the quality of your life.

4: Re-creating Yourself

What's the best way to improve your life? Assuming that you are past denying that it would be good for you to change, how can you most effectively and efficiently create a better you?

All I mean by 're-creating yourself' here is any deliberate action undertaken to produce a beneficial result in how you think, how you feel, or how you behave.

Why not learn from the successes and failures of others?

Imitation often works well. Find people who have the skill you want. Study them to find out how they think and act. Once you understand that, devise a plan that might work for you and train yourself to think and act their way. If it works, excellent. If it doesn't, investigate further to discover why it didn't work for you. Then create a revised plan and test it. Persist until success.

Psychologists have studied successful self-change and it'd be foolish not to consider their findings.[16] You may wonder, "Would I be better to hire some professional help rather than trying to change myself?"

In a sense, you already have – by obtaining this book.

If you are able to afford it, you might wonder about hiring a psychiatrist, clinical psychologist, or a consulting philosopher to help you.

Psychiatrists are physicians who specialize in studying and treating mental diseases. Unless you are mentally ill, you are not really a candidate for psychiatric treatment.

Clinical psychologists come from all kinds of schools of thought such as psychoanalytic, humanistic/existential, gestalt/experimental, cognitive, behavioral, NLP, and acceptance & commitment therapists. Rather than focusing on helping normal people live well, although there are some exceptions most clinical psychologists focus on helping people who are living poorly to live normally. So, unless you are sub-normal, hiring a clinical psychologist may not be very beneficial.

In North America, there are very few philosophers with a consulting practice.

(Personally, if I were in the market I would most seriously consider either a consulting philosopher or an acceptance & commitment therapist.)

Permit me four points about hiring someone to help you live better, more wisely.

First, successful self-change is possible. Indeed, throughout human history, that has been the most common way to improve. You don't need to hire someone to improve yourself.

(Incidentally, as a discipline separate from philosophy, psychology is a child of the Enlightenment and psychiatry originated in the latter part of the 19th century. There have been philosophers for at least two-and-one-half millennia.)

Second, successful self-change is not easy. Until new rituals are established, it requires persistent effort and attention. Since it is not easy, it often requires multiple attempts. Furthermore, the action required must be of an appropriate kind.

Third, hiring a consultant can be helpful. Understand, though, that a consultant is like a hired coach or friend. If you and the consultant are compatible and if you are willing to be accountable to your consultant, he or she may make persistent action easier. Furthermore, the consultant should be experienced in understanding the kind of action required, and, so, be able to guide your efforts. Still, again, nobody controls your attention but you—and that is the most critical element.

Fourth, your odds of success are equally good whether you opt for self-change or for hiring a consultant. (The important exception to this is if your brain is unhealthy. If it might be, hire a psychiatrist because they are also medical doctors.)

Whether you are working with a consultant or not, what should you do?

I don't know.

Nobody else knows, either. It's important that you understand why this is so. Permit me to explain it again.[17]

Whether you are working with a consultant or not, what should you do?

The critical concept here is the ordinary concept of evidence. When we lack evidence, we have no way to distinguish true from false judgments.

The traditional distinction between "knowledge" and "opinion" comes from dividing evidence into two sorts, namely, "demonstrative" evidence and "nondemonstrative" evidence. Knowledge is backed by demonstrative evidence and opinion is, or should be, backed by nondemonstrative evidence.

What's the difference?

Demonstrative evidence provides certainty. It's conclusive. It's indubitable. <u>Knowledge</u> is always true. Knowledge requires demonstrative evidence, which is evidence that makes mistake inconceivable.[18] So the extent of our knowledge is very limited. We can know, for example, present states (for example, "I have a headache") and simple conceptual truths (for example, "red is a color") but not much more.

On the other hand, every <u>opinion</u> is dubitable. If we only have "nondemonstrative" evidence, mistake is conceivable. We lack certainty. Even when we find them plausible or persuasive, opinions are always dubitable. It's always possible that an opinion is false.

When evaluating a judgment, it's important to determine whether it is known or whether it is an opinion. Is it possible to be mistaken in believing it? If so, it's not knowledge.

Despite what most people seem to think, perception, for example, is, notoriously, <u>not</u> a source of knowledge.[19] A perceptual judgment may be true, but it may also be false. Since it may be false, perception is not a source of knowledge.[20]

Why? Again, there's no such thing as false knowledge. Opinions, though, may be true or false. Any source of thoughts such as perception that only yields opinions is not a source of knowledge.

"Right" actions decrease suffering; "wrong" actions increase suffering. Right actions have good consequences that outweigh their bad consequences; wrong actions have bad consequences that outweigh their good consequences.

In general, what we would like is to engage in right actions so that we get the consequences, such as killing cravings, that we want. The important claim is this: there is no knowledge of which action would be right. Why? Given the difference between knowledge and opinion, the argument is simple:

Our actions (what we do) and inactions (what we do not do) have future consequences

It is senseless to evaluate actions as right or wrong without considering their consequences.

We are unable to know the future. We are unable to know the future consequences of any present actions or inactions.

Hence, we are unable to know whether a contemplated action is right or wrong.

That result certainly goes against what you were taught as a child, but it's really common sense. Everyone realizes that we are unable to predict the future, which is unknown and unknowable. (Still, we don't even like admitting that we may be mistaken.)

So, whenever we predict the future consequences of our actions or inactions, we may make a mistake. We may get it wrong. It is impossible to know the future; in fact, it's impossible to have *any* evidence about the future. It's important not to lie to ourselves; it's important not to pretend we know when we don't.

So let's have more humility. I don't know what you should do or not do to get whatever future consequences you want. Furthermore, nobody else has such knowledge either. All anyone has are opinions, which are really guesses based, at best, on nondemonstrative evidence.[21]

Understanding this is helpful for at least two important reasons.

First, if you have been beating yourself up for making mistakes, please stop. Mistakes are impossible to avoid. The human condition is to make decisions without knowing how they will turn out and then to enjoy or suffer whatever consequences occur (whether they are intended or not). Even sages make mistakes. After all, they, too, are human. If you did something or failed to do something that had terrible consequences, learn whatever lesson you are able to learn and let it go. Accept that you are not perfect and get on with your life.

Don Juan: "Challenges are simply challenges. The basic difference between an ordinary man and a warrior is that a warrior takes everything as a challenge, while an ordinary man takes everything as a blessing or a curse."

Second, please apply that same reasoning to others, too. They make mistakes. They are human. You don't have to take their mistakes personally. You don't have to keep blaming them for having made them. Let them go. Forgive others, too.

Also related to this is how bad we all are at *emotional estimation*. Very often someone will work very hard to achieve a certain goal with the expectation that he will live joyfully after having achieved that goal from then on. Think, say, of Olympic athletes who work for years and finally win a gold medal. Then what? They find that they do not live joyfully from then on. It works the same for you and me if we want a certain person as a lover, or we want a certain job, or we want a certain house, or we want a certain experience.

We are, in fact, notoriously bad at emotional estimation. Certain experiences generate positive emotions when we didn't expect them to, and certain other experiences, which we thought would be a source of continuing positive emotions, turn out not to be such a source.

The lesson is to become much more skeptical about predicting the future, especially future emotions.

Exercise 6

Please pause and consider this. Has it been true for you?

What is the best example from your own life of what you thought at the time was a bad event that turned out to have very unexpectedly good consequences? What is the best example from your own life of what you thought at the time was a good event that turned out to have very unexpectedly bad consequences?

Both have certainly happened to me repeatedly. Don't they happen to everyone? If so, it shows the importance of being skeptical about your own evaluations. It's best to subject them, too, to an attitude of detachment.

The primary reason why we are bad at emotional estimation is our amazing capacity for adapting to changed circumstances. It's important to consider *adaptability* whenever you are planning to make a change.

Here's a simple example. Suppose that you unexpectedly inherit $1000 and that, since you began and stuck to a new exercise program for the past 90 days, you want to reward yourself by spending the money on something that will make you feel happier. How should you spend it?

Since you've never had one and have heard good reports about them, you've been toying with the idea of buying a new high-definition or three-dimensional flat-screen television. On the other hand, you have not been out of town for six months and are tempted by a real change of pace such as a hiking and camping vacation in the mountains. Which alternative would be better at increasing how happy you feel?

Lacking any knowledge of future consequences, all you (or anyone) can do is to imagine that future connections will sufficiently resemble past connections.

Let's assume that your initial experiences with both the television and the vacation would be quite enjoyable. What will happen next?

After, say, a hundred days of watching it, would your enjoyment of watching your new television be anything close to as intensely enjoyable as it was the first day or two you had it? Of course not. You'll have adapted to it. It'll just be watching television.

This important phenomenon is sometimes called "the hedonic treadmill." It's why **incessantly gaining** additional **possessions won't make you happy**. You'll just quickly adapt to owning them and become dissatisfied again. Furthermore, if it's possible to gain X, it's also possible to lose X.

Whenever you find yourself suffering from "the someday syndrome," which is thinking, "If only I had X, I'd feel better," be careful. Even if you do feel better, that feeling will quickly fade. Unless you deliberately extend them, all emotions do.

As for the vacation, even if your enjoyment of it never stimulates you again to hike and camp in the mountains, you'll continue to remember it as having been a unique, enjoyable experience for as long as your memory lasts. In a sense, it will become part of yourself; you'll identify yourself as someone who successfully spent time in the mountains.

So, if you factor in adaptability, your best guess should be the vacation over the television.[22]

Now consider a loss instead of a gain. For example, how would you feel if you succeed in permanently freeing yourself from cravings? Well, for a while you might feel really good as you thought about their absence. Soon, though, you'd quietly adapt. Still, even without any continued positive emotional reinforcement, you would have evolved to a better quality of life in the sense that you would have freed yourself from an important affliction.

These examples suggest an interesting question: are losses actually better than gains? I invite you to wonder about that.

Our actions are always shots in the dark. If you think about it, this must be the case. Why? The world is in incessant flux.

There's no need to evaluate this. It'd certainly be foolish to take it personally. It's just a fact. It's just the way the world is. Accept it.

We simply cannot know that what worked well yesterday will work well today or that what works well today will work well tomorrow.

The world turns, and there's usually not much we can do about it. We are simply unable to know what will happen next. We live in *uncertainty*, which is why those who think they know the difference between right and wrong actions are wrong.

The world is full of fanatics desperately attached to their thoughts. Since they do not live examined (much less detached) lives, I hope you'll have compassion for them and try to show them the better way. Unfortunately, they go around endlessly bothering the rest of us.

Please notice how the idea of uncertainty goes with the idea that it's best to keep an open mind. If the world were not in incessant flux, presumably we'd have a lot more knowledge. It's because it is in incessant flux that we have so little knowledge.

You cannot know what to do to bring about the change you want. I cannot know what you should do either, nor is there anyone else who could know.

This may explain why you may be as effective at self-change as hiring a consultant would be.

Sorry, but I have no magic solution to the problem of re-creating yourself. There are no magical solutions.

Again, there's no need to evaluate that. It's just a fact. If you want to make a successful change, a lasting improvement, you must pay the full price of changing from within.

There's no way to know what will get better and what will get worse. The most mature attitude is not to attach yourself to hoping that life will get better. It's actually to adopt a middle way between optimism and pessimism, which are nothing but attitudes composed of thoughts.

The way to live wisely or well is to detach from all thoughts, especially from all evaluations, and to live without distraction in the present moment.

When we have a serious personal problem, the result is likely to be emotional distress. We don't feel good. We may be anxious or depressed. We may find it hard to like ourselves. Since there is no way to know how to cure it, we may naturally be confused and begin to feel hopeless. The situation is made worse if we suffer from food cravings or other kinds of cravings.

If you happen to be in emotional distress right now, what should you do?

Again, I don't know. I can, however, tell you what experience has taught me to do. Here's my general procedure. If it makes sense to you, test it.

First, I'd remind myself that there's nothing inherently wrong with me. I happen to believe that, just because I'm a normal human being, I have the capacity to live well. The present difficulty is not a reflection on me; it's nothing personal.

Second, I'd decide to do whatever it takes to feel better. I'd commit myself wholeheartedly to doing whatever is required. If, for example, I have to think outside the box and let go of some of my comfortable, familiar thoughts, so what? I'd rather change my mind than continue to suffer. I've done it before.

To decide not to change would be to quit on myself, to decide not to try to live better. For me as a philosopher, that would be intolerable.

Besides, if I do nothing, my emotional distress may only get worse. It's better to act now when I'm in less distress than when I get very depressed and perhaps even suicidal.

Third, I'd remind myself that my feeling better is good for others. In fact, improving myself in order to help others is often easier than improving myself to help myself, and that's particularly true if my self-esteem happens to be low.

Now what? Is there anything specific I could do?

I could begin by getting out of my own way.

I could start by not being defensive about my distress and those of my actions or inactions that may have caused it or contributed to it. I've developed some rituals that haven't served me well, but that's human.

What could I learn from others who have had the same problem and cured it? What did they come to understand that I don't yet understand?

I could vividly imagine the consequences of not changing, which would help me motivate myself to take whatever action is required.

I could ask if I have anyone who could help me. Maybe, for example, someone could help me identify my psychological defenses in order to enable me to let go of them. Do I have someone close to me who loves me? Is there a group I could join? Is there a consultant I could hire?

I realize that it's impossible to know which actions would be right to take, but which ones could I test that *might* work?

I do not believe that there is a separate, substantial self that is "me."[23] I believe that my decisions and actions create myself. If so, how could I create a better identity? What could I begin to do right now that would improve me from the inside out?

What self-talk program could I create that might work?

Am I crystal clear about exactly what I want? Is it worth achieving even if its beneficial emotional consequences quickly evaporate?

What benefits will the improvement bring? I should write them down and keep them handy for times of weakness.

When I don't feel like it, is there someone else I could do it for? Might a public commitment help?

Am I prepared to change? Have I learned what I need to understand? Have I devised a plan that may work well for me?

Since I want to avoid big mistakes, I want to take small steps. Successful small steps create large successful changes. Do I have a specific sequence of small steps in mind?

When should I begin? I don't want to wait more than a week to begin. I should pick a good starting time.

Have I built proper diet and exercise into my plan?

In order to make changing as easy as possible, am I planning to eat and to exercise well? How will it be realistic for me to continue to do so as I otherwise work to improve myself?

Have I built proper rest and relaxation (R & R) into my plan? Have I built in a regular practice such as meditation for deep relaxation and stress relief?

Have I improved my environment so that it supports me rather than hinders me? At least for now, have I let go of people who are afflicted with negative attitudes?

Have I built into my plan a system for giving myself little rewards as I make progress from each small step to the next?

Exercise 7

The purpose of this exercise is for you to draft your own initial plan. Beginning with Chapter 6, I present the method that I recommend for killing food cravings.

Instead of just blindly following what I suggest, this exercise is for you to think through and draft your own initial personal plan based on your self-understanding.

Please don't skip this exercise. Take your time with it and base it on your self-understanding. The better the plan you create now, the more value you will get from the following chapters.

In them I offer you my suggestions. If they strike you as better than your own, simply revise your plan appropriately; if they don't, don't.

Benjamin Franklin: "Failing to plan is planning to fail." He's right: using instrumental reason to plan prevents automatic failure in achieving goals.

If you answer the five following questions, you'll have a solid conceptual framework for evaluating the suggestions I make in the following chapters. Comparing your plan to mine will provide you with a written map of the road ahead.

In the context of improving the quality of your life by reducing or eliminating cravings, what is your most important problem or frustration? Write it down.

What difficulties are you experiencing that that problem is causing? Write them down.

Ideally, what is the outcome you'd like with respect to that problem? Write it down.

What benefits would that outcome bring you (and others around you)? Write them down.

Based on what you have just written, what is a sequence of small steps that might generate the outcome you want?

Amplify and revise what you have written by including your answers to the questions listed earlier in this chapter.

Permit me to stress the importance of this exercise. Also, again, please sit down in a quiet place with pen and paper and do it when your mind is fresh and clear. (The best time for me to do such exercises is first thing in the morning.) Spend at least half an hour writing out all your answers, but spend as much time as you need to do it as well as possible.

Once you've done it, you will have a plan that might actually work well to improve your life. That already separates you from the 95% of people who only have vague wishes for improvement. Good work!

Notice one real advantage of your plan: it's reusable! In the coming chapters you are going to examine and, probably, revise it. In the coming weeks and months you are going to implement it and, probably, revise it in accordance with the feedback you receive.

Once you have achieved your desired outcome with respect to cravings, you will also have given yourself a proven, written plan for evolving to your next stage.

How valuable might that be for the rest of your life?

Priceless.

Circumstances are in constant flux. Isn't it likely that sometime in the future you may begin to feel cramped and realize that you need further growth? When that occurs, you'll be prepared with a tested plan that can easily be adapted to work for you in that situation.

That, my friend, is real insurance.

Please, though, do not misunderstand: even following a sequence of plans like this is insufficient for wisdom, for living well. They can work to enable you to solve specific problems, but, ultimately, my hope for you is that you'll grow beyond their usefulness.

You see, plans like these themselves are thoughts. They are not just thoughtful in the sense that, by the time you have conceived it, revised it, tested it, and polished it, your plan will be the result of a lot of good thinking. The plan that results from that process will be written down and communicated in language. In that sense, it's a creature of language, and it's bound to language.

Ultimately, my hope for you is that you'll *grow even beyond the bounds of language.*

The way to do that is to practice regularly and properly doing exactly that. If you don't master a relevant practice, you will live the rest of your life bound by language and conceptual thinking.

It's only a very small percentage of adults who ever break the bonds of language. Of course, until you break those bonds by mastering a relevant practice, it's impossible to know whether the time and effort spent practicing will be worth it. It may be, or it may not be.

Until you directly experience such freedom for yourself, it can only be a matter of faith.

Minimally, it's important that you at least understand that you have that option. If you don't understand that it's even possible to live beyond the bounds of language, you'll not have the opportunity to decide for yourself whether or not to go for it. [See Chapter 11.] Meanwhile, why not wonder what growing beyond the bounds of language might be like?

Before we get there, however, let's begin to work towards greater freedom by working on your personalized plan to kill food cravings.

[SPECIAL OFFER SIDEBAR:

If the possibility of hiring a consulting philosopher interests you, I encourage you to have a look at my site at: http://www.ConsultingPhilosopher.com .

My suggestion is to click on the "Resources" tab at the top of the page and read the sections listed in its drop-down menu.

Also, check out "What To Do" at the top of the page and write out your answers to questions 8 – 28, which by themselves may help you gain insight on your own situation.

If you would like to speak privately with me one-on-one on the telephone for 15 minutes without paying for the consultation, contact me and mention this special offer from this book. There'll be no strings attached. If you would then like to hire me for a specific amount of time and I agree to accept you as a client, I'll give you a one-time whopping **50% DISCOUNT** on my consulting fee.]

5: Cultivation Before Seeding

It's normal to pay attention to what we are doing only a small fraction of the time. This is sufficient by it-self to account for why we don't feel good: most of the time our thoughts are separated from what we are doing. It's this nearly constant separation that fuels our nearly constant discontent, almost incessant dissatisfaction.

Walking was the example discussed previously. What goes for walking goes for nearly everything else we do.

On the other hand, we all do have the ability to pay attention. This happens to everyone in emergencies, which occasionally punctuate our everyday boredom.

Since the basic problem is that we tend to live in our heads, the basic solution is to train ourselves to stop doing that.

Exercise 8

You are an experienced adult. I hope that you have learned that it's impossible to get something for nothing. If you want anything of value, then you must give up something of value for it.

What are you willing to give up to free yourself from food cravings? More generally, what are you willing to give up to free yourself from all cravings?

What are you willing to trade to gain more opti-mal experiences? Instead of being stuck in ruts, what are you willing to give that will enable you more and more to enjoy a life that flows?

Write it down. That's the exercise.

Think of some sages. If you have never known one personally, think of ones you have read about or otherwise learned about.

Were they wealthy? It's not necessary to be financially wealthy to live wisely or well. It helps to be sufficiently wealthy so that all your basic needs (such as food, water, shelter, health care, social stability, and peace) are met. It's not easy to live well, and it's even more difficult in the midst of famine, drought, homelessness, sickness, social upheaval, or war.

For any normal North American reading this, being insufficiently wealthy to live well is not likely to be a problem. If you need more money, it's not that difficult to obtain it. (How? The basic plan is simple: Figure out what people want to buy. Match those demands to your aptitudes and skills. As long as the service or product you provide would benefit your customers, develop a product or service that works well, market and sell it for a profit.)

If it's not wealth that you will have to sacrifice for a significantly improved life, what will you have to sacrifice?

Time and focused effort.

I suggest <u>one hour daily of focused effort for the next six months</u>. Are you willing to do that? Could you give up, for example, an hour of television to focus on establishing rituals that will serve you a lot better for the rest of your life? Could you go to bed an hour earlier and get up an hour earlier in order to train?

If not, I'm pessimistic about your chances of ever succeeding. On the other hand, if you are willing to commit at least an hour daily (and an hour and a half would be even better), I'm optimistic about your chances.

Whatever amount of time and focused effort you are willing to commit, *write it down* in your daily planner. Note that there's no requirement that all your training occur in one clock hour; in fact, it may prove much better for you to break it up. As always, test the alternatives and see which one works best for you.

What does the training involve? There are only 6 steps. Once you learn what to do and begin practicing them for a few weeks, you'll see that they are all simple. They are all natural, too.

They are (1) taking better control of your eating, (2) taking better control of your fitness, (3) taking better control of your rest and recovery, (4) taking better control of your strength, (5) taking better control of your interpersonal encounters, and (6) taking better control of your mind.

In your initial enthusiasm, please do not try to improve everything all at once. Instead, it's very important to work on only one step at a time and, even then, only to take baby steps.

How long will each step take? That's up to you. Psychologists seem to agree that it takes at least 3 and 10 weeks to establish a new ritual. If so, don't tackle a new domain more frequently than every three weeks.

I suggest adding one ritual each month. If so, that means spending at least an hour daily for the next six months. If that pace is too rapid for you really to make them habitual, then I suggest adding the rituals involved in each step at a pace of one every two months.

The **goal**, then, is to have, at the end of six or twelve months, effective rituals established in all six areas.

Each of them is important. If you only took the first step, you would discover that you are much better off in a few months than you are today.

However, if you establish all 6, I predict that you are really, really going to be glad that you did after six months or a year. You are not going to have to wait that long to experience any benefits, but you are going to have to wait until you establish appropriate rituals in all

81

6 domains before you begin to experience all the benefits.

Because **each ritual is simple, natural, and sustainable,** there's no reason to begin by being in fear of the program. Instead, be excited! Here's a great opportunity to improve in a rational way what you may already be doing.

Consider, for example, eating. You have eating rituals established. The odds are that your percentage of body fat is too high. That means that the way you eat could be improved, and the improvements will be sustainable if they are well-conceived and implemented in a coherent manner that involves small steps.

Excess breeds failure. If you are serious about success, the 6 step method presented here should be implemented in small steps. The consequences of each of the small steps will probably be minor, not major. That's desirable. The feedback you receive from those minor steps will enable you, if necessary, to adjust what you are doing. If you proceed in that reasonable way, you'll soon find yourself far ahead, far from where you began.

Each small step, though, will require a burst of energy followed by sufficient recovery. In this way, the training is balanced.

If you train too hard for too long, you'll burn out and quit. If you fail to train hard enough or long enough, you won't see any benefits and you'll quit.

So there should be a balance between over-use and under-use, a middle way.

The way to train properly is to train wholeheartedly but intermittently: expend energy for a while and then renew energy for a while. This is done systematically. When you train hard and briefly, you'll push your limits, but then you'll allow for sufficient recovery before training hard again so that your capacity will increase.

A negative attitude will block you from training wholeheartedly. If you suffer from one, you'll always be holding yourself back.

For example, in doing research on diabetes,[24] I was recently reading a book in which the author correctly extolled the benefits of strength training because it in-increases muscle mass. That's important if you are trying to prevent your blood glucose[25] levels from going too high because muscles are the tissues that use the most glucose. Then she writes that she herself does strength training and finds it "dull." It's her negative attitude that makes strength training dull for her! I've done strength training for many years and taught others how to do it. Done properly, which means intensely with perfect exercise technique, it is anything but dull. I wouldn't want anyone with her attitude training with me.

Training without intense focus fails. Overly enthusiastic unbalanced training also fails.

Brief, intense training that intermittently balances energy expenditure with energy renewal succeeds.

If you understand that, you already understand how to train. Train intensely and briefly while ensuring that you obtain plenty of thorough rest.

If you also understand why working on establishing different improvements one at a time is better than trying to change everything simultaneously, you are ready to avoid training that is counterproductive. However, that insight invites the question: what's the best sequence for establishing the six kinds of rituals?

I don't know your best sequence. However, it is probably the sequence as I present it in the following chapters. Why? The general justification has already been mentioned, namely, it's impossible or very difficult to live wisely or well with an unhealthy brain and body. If you were to attempt, for example, gaining better control of your emotions or of your power of focus while being in poor physical condition, you would have far more difficulty and experience less success than otherwise.

Exercise 9

Slip into your best clothes, your best suit or dress if you have one. Stand in front of a full-length mirror and have a good look at yourself. Do you look pretty good?

Then undress and stand naked in front of that mirror. Question: are you looking at someone who might be able to survive in the wild as a successful hunter and gatherer?

If you are like most of the rest of us, you are not. In other words, you look physically unlike your successful Stone Age ancestors.

So let's change that. Let's initially ensure that you are eating, exercising, and recovering well physically.

If you happen already to be in excellent physical condition, you'll sail through the first several steps with, perhaps, just a few minor adjustments in your rituals.
If you are normal and not already in excellent physical condition, you'll need to make significant changes but, also, you'll quickly begin to experience some of the major benefits of this method, which will increase your motivation to work though all 6 steps.

It is important to have the blessing of your personal physician before making any significant changes in your dietary or exercise habits. It's only on the basis of a thorough physical exam, which may reveal anomalies, that your physician should advise you. So please don't execute even the initial steps of this program until you get a go-ahead from your medical doctor.

For example, it's possible that, although you don't know it, you have developed type-2 diabetes and the physical exam by your physician reveals that. A normal blood sugar is about 83 or 85 mg/dl and your exam revealed, let us suppose, a significantly higher level. What has happened is that your body has lost at least part of its ability to compensate when your blood sugar level is either too high or too low.

So, to avoid the debilitating and sometimes deadly consequences of having blood sugar levels that are out of control, since it's not possible to cure diabetes, you now realize that you need to assist your body by taking over, with the assistance of modern medical technology, for the automatic capacity it lost. Your new task is to learn how to normalize blood sugar levels and incorporate those changes into your personalized 6-step plan.

The plan I present assumes that you are perfectly healthy. Is anyone really perfectly healthy? Whether detected yet or not, we all probably have some physical anomalies.

Furthermore, if you are addicted to any recreational drugs such as nicotine, alcohol, or cocaine, it's important to break those addictions if you genuinely value your health.

Even if you don't have any such addictions and are lucky, you will grow old and eventually get sick and die. If you are not lucky, you will die long before you grow old. Either way, that's humiliating, isn't it? We'd like to have much more control over our destinies than that. Shedding that feeling permanently is yet another reason for regular spiritual, as well as physical, training. [I return to this in Chapter 11.]

If you already know that you have certain abnormalities, after consultation with your physician, simply incorporate them into your personalized plan. On the other hand, if you don't appear to have any, just continue to get regular screenings and be alert for any that develop.

In this case, to continue with the same example, if you are diabetic you should wait at least 3 or 4 hours after a meal before eating again (unless you are injecting insulin in which case you should wait at least 5 hours after a meal before eating again). In other words, personalize the plan by modifying it to suit your individual circumstances.

I am able to keep my presentation of the plan as simple as possible only by assuming that it is for completely healthy people.

There's simply **no one way that works best for everyone**. I present this method with the expectation that you will use it only when the tactics I suggest make more sense for you than the tactics in your own plan, which you should already have in writing.

It may still surprise you (and your physician) that the plan I recommend really does work for promoting excellent health as well as for living wisely. This is not actually so surprising once you realize that being healthy and living wisely are similar in that they both centrally involve *dynamic resiliency*. It's not that excellent health means never getting sick; instead, excellent health means being able to recover physical well-being rapidly after it has been lost. Similarly, it's not that living wisely means never getting knocked off balance; instead, it means being able to recover balance rapidly after it has been lost. Living wisely is centered living.

With respect to justification, it would be impossible for me to cite all the evidence I have accumulated over the years in favor of the 6 specific steps that I recommend. However, where there is widespread confusion, especially about what it means to eat well [in the next chapter], I do briefly give reasons for my recommendations. More extensive justifications are readily available on my websites, my blog, my other books, and in the books and other resources by others listed in the Selected Bibliography, and elsewhere.

If you alter what I suggest and find that your way works well, excellent. If you find, however, that your altered way fails to work as well as you had hoped, please don't quit. Just go back to my recommendation and try that.

I've personally made lots of mistakes. For example, I was a vegetarian for about a decade and tried to be healthy and lean on a high carb diet. I failed. (I stayed too fat.) For example, I tried to live wisely for decades without having a spiritual practice. I failed. (I crashed emotionally.) For example, I tried strength training every day. I failed. (I became weaker.) And so on.

Everyone makes mistakes. It's important to learn from them and to keep mistakes as small as possible.
I want you to avoid my mistakes. This method just isn't based on reading a lot in the relevant areas (although I've done that); it's also based on my direct experience. These are the best suggestions I have.[26]

The 6-step method presented in the following chapters is a *natural* one—and, therefore, it may require significant changes to your self-image. If so, make them *before* you begin using the plan.

By "natural" I mean one that your successful ancestors of 20,000 or 50,000 years ago could have utilized to enjoy and enhance well-being.

It's true that nobody today knows exactly what they were like. Like us, they were not all the same; they had different (though primitive) cultures and inhabited different regions of the earth. However, scientists have pieced together enough nondemonstrative evidence that enables us to have considerable confidence that our understanding of what they were like is correct.

The fact is that your ancestors were successful hunters, fishermen, and gatherers. They looked the part, too. As a group, they were fitter, stronger, leaner, and healthier than we are. (Furthermore, many even had more leisure time than we do.) Why is there that difference? It's because we have been debilitated as individuals by many of the advances of civilization.

The critical physical fact to absorb is that their bodies were almost identical to ours. It's true that evolution is still going on, but it's also true that at least 99.9% of our genes are exactly the same as theirs were. **At least physiologically, civilization has made us worse off than our Stone Age ancestors.** That means that we've done it to ourselves – and there's no reason we cannot improve our condition by rediscovering what we evolved to do.

The genetic changes that have occurred since the first agricultural revolution have been very minor. For example, they never consumed dairy products whereas, even as an adult, you may be able to digest the lactose (milk sugar) they contain with little apparent difficulty. Except for human breast milk, they never drank milk (imagine trying to harvest milk from wild mammals like antelope or buffalo!) whereas you may drink as much as a quart of cow's milk daily. They never ate breakfast cereals, breads, or pastas whereas you may get the majority of your calories from carbohydrates. They never drank beer, wine, or spirits whereas you may consume them regularly.

Also, of course, they were much more active than we are. They had to walk or jog to reach distant locations whereas you and I are able to drive or fly to them while seated. If you have ever done any real camping in wilderness, you know that it involves physically hard work. They lived on a perpetual camping trip.

New behaviors such as consuming dairy products, lots of processed (refined) carbohydrates, and alcoholic beverages that are instituted and passed down through the generations can, and have, spawned minor genetic changes. Sometimes, these changes can be very important to certain individuals.

However, on the whole these changes are very minor. For context, we still share over 98% of our genetic code with the pygmy chimp of Zaire and the common chimpanzee, who are our closest living relatives. The genetic changes between you and one of your ancestors 20,000 years ago are so modest that they are almost insignificant.

If you really do understand that it's impossible to gain anything of value for nothing, then you are in a good position to understand how certain cultural advances such as the first agricultural revolution (farming, the domestication of plants), the domestication of animals (ranching), the development of literacy, and the mechanization of work can be blessings for civilization and yet also be curses for individuals.

For example, individuals can become addicted to consuming dairy products, carbohydrates, and alcoholic beverages. Such addictions can have serious negative consequences on physical and mental well-being. Furthermore, we civilized humans have the option of developing insidious habits such as being attached to reading, physical inactivity, or incessant conceptualization that also undermine well-being and also were not options for our ancestors. That's the bad news.

The good news is that we, unlike them, also have **the option of maximizing the benefits of civilization while minimizing the liabilities of civilization on us as individuals**.

That's the fundamental perspective behind the simple 6-step method presented in the following chapters.

Ovid: "Let others praise ancient times, I am glad to be alive in these."

Let's assume that you have not already established the rituals associated with the 6 steps of this method and that, where necessary, you will personalize the plan to fit your individual circumstances. I contend that, if you will incorporate the rituals associated with a single step – one step at a time -- into your life for the

89

next six (or twelve) months, you are going to experience *an overall surge of well-being* that will astound you.

Furthermore, each time you savor a benefit from using your plan, you are going to be that much more motivated to continue improving in accordance with it.

Why shouldn't your life continue to improve until your dotage?

I contend that, if you install the appropriate rituals from your personalized plan over the next six (or twelve) months and continue with them, you will be maximizing the chances for that to occur.

Right now, it's only a matter of faith. In a few short months, there should be no need for you to have that faith anymore. You'll have directly experienced vastly enhanced well-being for yourself. The faith will have been replaced by your own experience.

To put the greatest odds of success in your favor, if you don't already, from a physical point of view begin thinking of yourself as a successful hunter and gatherer. Imagine that you were just living your life 20,000 years ago and were abruptly fast-forwarded into the 21st century. How should you behave to sustain your physical well-being?

You don't have to look far to find the answer: you should behave in terms of eating and exercising much as today's natural fitness models and bodybuilders behave. ('Natural' here denotes those from those two groups who do not use drugs such as anabolic steroids to enhance their physiques.) There are physical role models of both sexes and all ages available for you to emulate.[27]

I encourage you to learn how to flourish physically from studying past role models (your anscestors) and present role models (natural fitness models and bodybuilders). If you do, the physical rituals you'd come up with will be quite similar to the ones I recommend in what follows.

I've done the work for you.

By all means, however, be skeptical of what I recommend and do the research for yourself. (Though I doubt you will, I'd certainly appreciate your telling me if you come up with anything significantly different than what I recommend for a healthy, normal person.)

Ready to enhance your physical well-being? Ready to begin to flourish more physically?

That's not all there is to living well, but the other rituals all depend upon physical ones.

A final reminder about attitude before you begin the 6 steps: make "**UUM**" your new mantra. *Understand. Use. Modify.*

You'll understand the 6 steps by understanding the following chapters. Then, if they make sense to you, take those steps. Make adjustments based on the feedback you receive and continue to use them.

Personalize the plan so it works well for you. If you then work your plan, it will work well for you.

6: Taking Better Control of Your Eating

Ancient Greeks would visit the oracle at Delphi seeking her prophecy. There were two maxims posted above the entrance to her chamber. They translate as "Know Thyself" and "Nothing In Excess."

There's much wisdom in those maxims. Please keep them in mind as you learn the 6 steps of The Killing Cravings Method. Ignore them at your peril. Successfully implementing the first step, the plan for eating well presented in this chapter, depends upon both maxims.

Here's what will happen: once you begin eating well and allow your body a few days to adjust to your new diet, 90% of your food cravings will vanish – never to return as long as you continue eating well. In that sense, this first of the 6 steps is the most important.

Do you think that your successful ancestors lived to eat, or do you think that they ate to live?

I think they ate to live, and you would be wise to follow their example.

You want to get off to a fast start, right?

If so, assuming you aren't already following them, immediately improve how you eat in accordance with the guidelines presented in this chapter.

That's your chief task for the next month (or two). It's your only task. You don't even need to finish reading the next chapter in this book until the beginning of next month.

Whatever else happens in your life this month, if you do that you are going to be able to look back and remember this month as the month that your life began to get better and better. Let's get your life spiraling upward rather than downward.

Except dissatisfaction, what do you have to lose?

Depending upon what you are already doing, the first three days in particular may be difficult as your body switches from burning sugar to burning fat. However, with your initial enthusiasm intact just resolve to blast through them. If you've been eating a normal North American diet, you will be able to measure progress in a few days and, even by the end of the first week, you may already feel quite proud of what you have accomplished.

Frequency

Eat (3 or) 4 times during the day.

If you select a 4X nutrition plan, you'll be having a meal about every 4 waking hours, which is similar to what many people do anyway.

A calorie is nothing but a measure of the energy (heat) provided by foods. It's the amount of energy it takes to raise the temperature of 1 milliliter of water 1 degree C.

If you ingest more calories than you expend, you'll gain body fat; if you ingest fewer calories than you expend, you'll lose body fat. So what is required is to find the middle way that works best for you between too few calories and too many calories.

It's important to avoid the <u>common dieting mistake</u> of getting **too few** calories. Whether you are male or female, large or small, **never** allow your total daily calories to go below 2000 cal. Why?

According to the World Health Organization, anything less than that is a starvation diet. In the long run, not only are starvation diets unhealthy, but also they don't work for lasting weight loss.

Many popular fad diets are starvation diets. Partly because you may have been bombarded with advertisements for them, you may have tried them. If so, you probably already realize that, although they may work for a while to reduce body weight, as soon as you go off them, you find yourself actually worse off than before you started. They are counterproductive physically as well as being discouraging.

Why?

Here are four important relevant facts.

First, muscle is many times metabolically more active than fat. A pound of muscle may metabolize (burn, beta oxidize) several dozen times more calories in the same time as a pound of fat.

Second, what counts is not your body weight but your body fat percentage. Your body fat percentage is the amount of fatty tissue you have relative to the amount of muscle and other tissue you have. You may be, statistically, of "normal" weight but still too fat. Is your percentage of body fat 30% or 15%? There's a very big difference.

(What should be your percentage of body fat? That's a question for you to answer. 15% would be a very good percentage if you are a woman, and 10% would be a very good percentage if you are a man.[28])

Third, muscle tissue is denser than fatty tissue. A pound of muscle takes up less volume than a pound of fat. This explains why – even though they may look smaller -- trim fitness models, strength trainers, and athletes with a relatively low percentage of body fat can weigh more than people with a higher percentage of body fat.

Fourth, when we lose body weight through starvation diets, we lose about half muscle tissue and half fatty tissue.

Suppose that you go on a starvation diet, lose 20 pounds of body weight, and, when you go off the diet, you regain it. How could you be physically worse off than before you began the diet?

It's because the regained body weight will be almost all fatty tissue. Even though your body weight before and after the whole episode was the same, your body composition would be worse afterwards because you would have lost about 10 pounds of muscle.

If you have gone through this cycle multiple times, your body composition is much worse than it used to be. In effect, you worked hard by forcing yourself to stick to a starvation diet for a while, eventually you went off it, and, sadly, you wound up worse off than you were before you began, and you repeated that discouraging process more than once.

What's the important takeaway lesson here?

First, never diet! Although they seem good in theory, reducing diets based on counting calories don't work. [See the next section.] Instead, make only changes that you can live with for the rest of your life. Take small steps. Nothing in excess.

In addition to eating more naturally, which is the topic of this chapter, the other steps of The Killing Cravings Method should also be used regularly for the rest of your life. Used in conjunction with each other, the 6 steps will almost certainly enable you to achieve and maintain a healthful body composition. If you need to lose body fat, they will enable you to achieve a much better body composition in a way that is sustainable.

That will enable you to look better, feel better, have a much healthier percentage of body fat, and be more energetic.

So forget about weighing your body. If you lost 10 pounds of fatty tissue and gained 10 pounds of muscle tissue, your body would weigh the same but your percentage of body fat would be significantly improved. Instead, once a week measure your percentage of body fat.[29] Why? It's easier to improve what can be measured than it is to improve what cannot be measured.

Keep energy consumption roughly the same at each meal. Do not, for example, eat 4 tiny meals and then 1 huge meal for dinner. If, using a 4X, 5X, or 6X nutrition plan, you begin consuming nutrients in a more evenly, this one adjustment alone may enable you to feel better. A more even intake of nutrients will, by itself, reduce blood sugar spikes, mood swings, and food cravings.

It is not, however, just the frequency of your meals that matters: it's also, and especially, what you eat.

Food Count Content

Not all calories are equal.

It's useful to think in terms of the three kinds of macronutrients in foods, namely, fats, proteins, and carbohydrates (carbs).

Natural fats should be the chief source of your daily calories. Get about one-third of your calories from proteins. Get the small remained of your calories from carbs.

Since natural sources of proteins include fats, the same food sources will give you both fats and proteins. They naturally go together. Those sources should constitute most of what you eat.

Relating this to real foods is complicated. Abstractly, a gram of dietary fat has about 9 calories, a gram of alcohol has about 7 calories, and a gram of either dietary carbohydrate or dietary protein has about 4 calories.

However, real foods are concrete, not abstract. Your body expends more energy getting the energy from dietary fat and dietary protein than from dietary carbohydrate. The net energy available from dietary fat is about 5 (rather than 9) calories a gram. The net energy available from an ounce (28.5 grams) of dietary protein is only about 6 grams.

Assuming that you are healthy and also following the other 5 steps, I recommend eating natural foods and keeping in mind just *two general guidelines*.

First, get sufficient protein at each meal, preferably from natural sources.

How much is that? Simply divide your lean body weight by the number of your meals. For example, if you weigh 200 pounds, your lean body weight is 140, and you adopt a 4X plan, consume on average about 35 grams of protein per meal.

This is minimum requirement. If you do heavy physical work or serious strength training, you'd be wise to increase it.[30] A traditional method is to divide your body weight in pounds by the number of meals in order to obtain the average number of grams of protein per meal. (Some large bodybuilders ingest 300 to 500 grams of protein daily.) This will help prevent your body going into starvation mode and lowering its metabolic rate and ensure that you are ingesting both essential amino acids and essential fatty acids. To say that they are essential is to say that our bodies cannot make them; we must get them from our diet. Given how our bodies evolved, this is perfectly natural.

On the other hand, if you are struggling to lose body fat and following one of these guidelines, you may go slightly below these minimum protein requirements temporarily until you reach your target percentage of body fat.

Second, consume no more than 25 grams of carbs nearly every day and spread that consumption among your 4 meals.

Especially if you are pre-diabetic or diabetic, 25 is the maximum number.

Even though this comes as part of the first step, it may well be *the single most difficult improvement required for killing food cravings.*

If you have ever tried measuring portion sizes and counting calories, you will immediately realize how much easier these two guidelines are to follow than doing that. Yes, for a week or two you will probably need to rely on some food counts source.[31] However, except occasionally, you thereafter won't have to consult anything. Again, this is a natural diet; it's the diet your body evolved to eat. It's simple.

If you are afraid of fats and these recommendations shock you, that's understandable. If you think you should be getting most of your calories from carbohydrates, that, too, is understandable. All kinds of confused and confusing advice about what to eat has been proliferated for decades.

Carbs and proteins are the dietary sources of glucose. It's helpful to understand something about how they work.

Carbs are made of sugars. Chemically long chains of sugars are "polysaccharides" ("many sugars") but they can't be absorbed by the intestines even when they are broken down in two sugar units ("disaccharides"). Enzymes must break them down to simple sugars ("monosaccharides") for absorption to occur. So all dietary carbs become simple sugars before they are used by the body. The only difference is that polysaccharides and disaccharides are absorbed more slowly than simple sugars.

Sugar delights us because it fosters neurotransmitter production (principally serotonin) in the brain, which relieves anxiety and makes us feel good and, even, euphoric. (Neurotransmitters are the chemical messengers the brain uses for communication.) This is why carbs are addictive to people whose brains are sensitive to, or depleted of, these neurotransmitters.

When blood sugar levels are low, the body can convert proteins into glucose. Thus dietary carbs are not essential, in other words, <u>dietary carbohydrates are unnecessary.</u> Given how our bodies evolved, getting a high percentage of calories from dietary carbs is unnatural.

Aldous Huxley: "Facts do not cease to exist just because they are ignored." Jean Martin Charcot: "Theories, no matter how pertinent, / Cannot eradicate the existence of facts."

Furthermore, dietary protein has a slower and smaller blood sugar effect than dietary carbohydrate and, because the process is not very efficient, the body has to work harder to do it.

The body cannot convert fat into sugar (nor can it convert glucose back into protein).

Your body uses an insulin-sensitive enzyme to burn fat. When you consume dietary carbs, if you are healthy your body will produce insulin in proportion to the amount of carbs you consumed. As your insulin levels increase, fat ozidation decreases.

I   n addition, glucose is the carbon backbone of carbs. Increased insulin signals your liver to convert glucose to fat, which is detectable in your blood as triglycerides, that gets stored. Bottom line: *the more carbss you consume, the fatter you will become.*

Where does body fat come from for most North Americans? It doesn't come from dietary fats; it comes from dietary carbs.

It does this using insulin, which is the main fat-building and fat-storing hormone. If you are slim and fit, you are probably very sensitive or responsive to insulin. The more abdominal fat you have (and also, though to a lesser degree, the more total body fat you have) compared to your lean body (muscle) mass, the less sensitive or responsive to insulin you will tend to be.

Since it's unnatural, it makes sense that the more insulin resistant you are, the more unhealthy you are.

The good news is that, for most people, insulin resistance can be reversed.

The way to reverse it is to consume fewer dietary carbs, to lose body fat, and to normalize blood sugar levels. In a healthy person, blood sugar levels after eating a meal do not spike. If your blood sugar levels spike after a meal, like skin discoloration from too much sun, it's a sign you are hurting yourself.

These ideas should build on what you already understand. For example, suppose you were a rancher and wanted to fatten up your pigs or cows for slaughter. What macronutrient would you feed them? Would you feed them lots of protein from eggs and meats, would you feed them lots of carbs from grains, or would you feed them lots of fats?

In fact, ranchers fatten them using grains—for good reason.

Perhaps, though, you should feed them fat? No. Fat will be converted to body fat but only if it is part of a high-carb diet. If it is part of a low-carb diet, it will be metabolized.

Similarly, if you want to reduce your percentage of body fat or keep it low, eat fats and proteins and don't eat carbs. It's simple.

If you need to open your mind and let some bad ideas escape, just do so. How?

You may need to modify the way you think of yourself.

Keep it simple. Remind yourself how your successful ancestors evolved to eat. Remind yourself how successful natural fitness models and bodybuilders (and many others who, like movie stars, emulate them) eat.

For example, your successful ancestors had no farms to produce wheat, corn, rice, or other grains. That means they consumed no foods made out of grains such as breads, pasta, pastries, rolls, muffins, crumpets, bagels, pretzels, cookies, cakes, corn chips, breakfast cereals, and so on.

They also had no flocks of cattle to produce dairy products. Imagine trying to milk wild buffalo or antelope! That means they did not consume milk, butter, yogurt, frozen yogurt, ice cream or cheese.

Since they didn't grow sugar cane, beets, corn, or other plants that we use to make sweeteners, they ate no candy, soda, sweet desserts, or any other foods sweetened with sugar. Except for honey, they never ate nutrient-null (empty) calories.

They ate very little or no salt.[32]

Since they had no canning or refrigeration, they never consumed any canned or frozen foods. Similarly, they didn't know how to mill or irradiate foods.

Since they weren't ranchers, they never consumed flesh foods from cattle or bison that were feed corn (instead of grass), pumped with antibiotics and hormones, and raised in crowded feedlots. At least until they domesticated dogs, they never ate the flesh of domesticated animals—and there are important differences between the flesh of domesticated animals and the flesh of wild animals. For example, there is less fat in the muscles of wild animals.

They did eat plant foods, but there are important differences between wild plant foods and cultivated plant foots. The wild plant foods they ate were smaller (and uglier) than what we have available in grocery stores. Wild plant foods have more protein, fiber, and calcium than cultivated plants while having less sugar and starch. (Sugars are sweet, water soluable carbohydrates that are monosaccharides or disaccharides. Starches are carbohydrate foods composed of long chains of glucose.)

They never ate processed foods. They didn't have some of our modern plant foods (like corn) and the ones they had were dissimilar to their descendants that are available to us many, many, many plant generations later. Remember that almost all the modern plant foods we eat critically depend upon using fertilizers, pesticides, preservatives, and irrigation – none of which our successful ancestors had.

Their staple food came from the muscles, organs, and fat of wild game animals. Some of the fat of such animals, such as the bone marrow from large leg bones, was the most prized portion of the carcass.

They did, of course, learn to cook food. The purpose of cooking is to break down foods so that their nutrients are more easily consumed.

They successfully hunted and fished and scavenged and gathered lots of different kinds of foods. They ate flesh foods from a wide variety of wild animals including animals that we rarely or never see in our grocery stores such as seal, whale, walrus, bear, antelope, cape buffalo, mammoth, many kinds of wild fish, snakes and other reptiles, squirrels and other small mammals, rodents, seeds, nuts, berries, wild fruits, eggs, wild vegetables, insects, tubers, and so on.

Yes, they were uncivilized. They had no modern medical or surgical science. They had no dentists. They had no writing or universities. They had no air conditioning or automobiles. Their art was primitive. They were superstitious and ignorant. We have many blessings they didn't have.

However, don't feel too sorry for them about their physical condition. Since our ancestors were the longest lived mammals on earth, their daily risk of death was small. In many physical environments such as sub-Saharan Africa, adults probably only "worked" 20 or 30 hours weekly. There were no epidemics or pandemics. There were no large-scale wars.

Although the domestication of plants and animals has given us plentiful food, the food it has produced is less reliable and less healthy than the food our ancestors had. Farming has made the grains and other plants we rely on less diverse, less nutritionally valuable, and less hardy. Ranching has made the animals we rely on less diverse, less nutritionally valuable, and less hardy.

Furthermore, living in close proximity to animals has given us humans some of the most serious infectious diseases we have ever encountered such as smallpox, measles, bird flu, tuberculosis, and AIDS.

The domestication of plants and animals has also created higher infant mortality for us, reduced our stature, and caused iron deficiency, bone disorders, chronic anemia, and poor dental health. It has also shortened our lifespan.

I recall wondering as a boy going to the dentist about how my Stone Age ancestors long ago dealt with cavities without dentists. As a boy whose father was a physician, I couldn't image how they survived without modern medications or surgical interventions. I just didn't get it.

If this way of thinking about macronutrients isn't familiar to you, I encourage you to do your own research. In just the last decade or two, more and more scientists, historians, and others have been waking up to the fact that there's been no free lunch. *The blessings of civilization have come at a high cost to many individuals.*

Christian B. Allan, Ph.D., and Wolfgang Lutz, M.D.: "Humans have evolved and are adapted to eat a diet of mostly animal fat and protein . . . carbohydrates are to a large extent responsible for most human illness." Kilmer S. McCully, M.D.: "The so-called 'diseases of Western civilization' – heart disease, obesity, hypertension, diabetes, cancer, dental caries, and others – became pervasive in human populations of developed nations during the twentieth century primarily because of the consumption of a diet containing refined carbohydrates . . ." Philip J Goscienski, M.D.: "All the chronic diseases of modern life are avoidable . . . most modern humans kill themselves, not by outright suicide but by the lifestyle they choose . . ." Loren Cordain, Ph.D.: "we are genetically adapted to eat what the hunter-gatherers ate. Many of our health problems today are the direct result of what we do – and do not – eat . . . The Paleo Diet is the one and only diet that ideally fits our genetic makeup. Just 500 generations ago – and for 2.5 million years before that – every human on Earth ate this way."

Once someone points it out, like all great ideas the idea of **eating mostly natural fats and proteins** to promote good health is simple.

Once you really get it, you'll easily be able to make food choices that are likely to serve you much, much better than the food choices you've been making. It if has a food label, think twice before consuming it.

The chief guideline is very simple: **before putting food into your mouth, ask if your successful ancestors 20,000 years ago could have eaten it (or a food very similar to it). If not, don't eat it**. This test will always give you immediate practical help cutting through confusion and hype.

On the other hand, if you've been ingesting 300 grams of carbs daily and cut down to 25, that will require some major adjustments to what you eat. There are, though, no excuses: if you want the benefits, just make the adjustments. You'll be delighted you did.

In measuring carbs, count only "net" carbs. In food count tables on packaging, some ingredients such as fiber have to be listed as carbs even though they have no effect at all on blood sugar levels. Just subtract them from the total carbs listed to get the net carbs.

It's worth noting that the Food and Drug Administration in the United States permits processed food manufacturers to be in compliance with the law if the figures they list on food packages are within 20% of the actual food counts. In other words, what is actually in a package is not necessarily what it says on the package. If you are concerned about that, just test yourself to see if a certain food spikes your blood sugar levels.[33]

The critical aspect of this first step is permanently cutting dietary carbs *each no more than 4 or 5 grams of carbs per meal.* Always avoid fast-acting carbs.

Instead, eat plenty of fats and proteins from natural sources such as grass-fed ungulates like beef, bison, or beefalo; wild caught seafood; game animals; uncaged poultry; eggs from uncaged chickens; and (preferably organic) low carb vegetables.[34]

The key to improving and sustaining the improvements is how you think. Please focus on the fact that you don't need any dietary carbs to be healthy.

Still, because of the phytonutrients and fiber they contain, it's a good idea to consume several servings of low-carb vegetables daily. Especially important are leafy green vegetables like spinach. Others are asparagus, lettuce, mustard greens, beet greens, turnip greens, parsley, kale, collard, bok choy, broccoli, cauliflower, celery, cucumber, cabbage (whether green, red, or Chinese), mushrooms, sweet or hot peppers, yellow summer squash and zucchini. Additionally, there are other natural foods, such as walnuts, that are permissible. (I eat some nuts, broccoli, red pepper, and raw organic spinach nearly every day.)

Avoid fruits and fruit juices. If you really like fruits and can afford the carbs, limit yourself to small quantities of (preferably organic) berries.

Learn about the psychology of eating well and put it to work for you. How? The main idea in this context is what always matters: pay attention to what you are doing. [I discuss this further in Chapter 11.]

I've been a philosopher since 1964. My considered opinion is that Gotama was the greatest sage of all time. Interestingly, he said something about eating well that reminds us of the two maxims at Delphi:

"When a man is always mindful, Knowing moderation in the food he eats, His ailments then diminish: He ages slowly, guarding his life."[35]

As usual, he's right on the mark. To eat well, always be mindful of what you are eating.

If you begin with self-understanding, if you begin by understanding how your mind actually works, you will make eating well as easy as possible for yourself.

If you want to be as kind as possible to others, begin by being as kind as possible to yourself.

For example, suppose that you are used to having a sweet dessert after meals. What should you do to have something sweet while not spiking your blood sugar with a high carb dessert? I discussed adaptability in Chapter 4. Why not use that to your advantage? Because we quickly adapt to a new taste, it's always the first taste of something that is the best Here's a tactic I often use: when I want something sweet at the end of a meal, I take one or two frozen organic strawberries from a bag in the freezer, run them under warm water for a moment, and pop them into my mouth. Their icy sweetness does the trick.

Here are some more helpful tips that work because they are based on sound psychology:

Never stand up when eating. Always eat in silence – otherwise conversation, music, and sounds from artificial sources such as televisions or radios will almost certainly distract you. *Instead of continuing to eat until you feel full, stop eating when you are no longer hungry.* Chew thoroughly and eat slowly in order to allow your body time to send out satiation signals. Avoid eating family style; instead, put everything you intend to eat on a plate before you begin eating. Be wary of visual illusions and use, for example, tall, skinny glasses, small dishes, and small spoons. Since they can stimulate cravings, avoid food odors like cinnamon buns and other freshly baked pastries. Always eat in the same place.

These are just a few examples of small adjustments you can make that will make it much easier to eat better.[36]

Martin Seligman, Ph.D.: "you can make major changes all throughout adulthood if you know the ways of changing that actually work . . . Growth and change are the rule, not the exception, throughout adult life."

That's true, isn't it? Like or not, we actually experience incessant flux. Why not embrace it? Fighting reality is always a losing battle. Why not take charge of it and turn the changes that we experience anyway into opportunities to enjoy life more?

We've seen how changing your self-image is critical. Start thinking of yourself as what you really are, namely, a successful descendant of successful hunter-gatherers.

Start thinking of some civilized foods as what they really are, namely, dangerous to your health and unnecessary. Since, when digested, all carbohydrates become simple sugars, think of a potato as a lump of sugar. Begin to "see" a loaf of bread as a block of sugar. If you practice deliberately thinking about such ubiquitous foods in such new ways and associating carbs with body fat, which is ugly, you'll diminish the temptation to put them into your mouth.

Many people who are too heavy are addicted to carbs. How can you tell if you are addicted to carbs?

It is impossible even for the best scientists to predict accurately how a certain food will behave in a certain individual. If you are healthy and not addicted to carbs, you should have a mean of about 83 to 85 milligrams of glucose per deciliter of blood. You can test your own blood or get it tested.

Assuming you are neither sick nor dehydrated, the causes of insulin resistance are inheritance, obesity, and high blood sugars. You cannot control your inheritance, but you can control obesity and high blood sugars.

Impaired fasting glucose is considered by many physicians to be a pre-diabetic condition. If you have fasting blood sugars over 99 mg/dl, the World Health Organization says that you have impaired fasting glucose. If you are pre-diabetic and do not permanently eat as recommended here, it is probably only a matter of time before you develop diabetes.

Obesity plays a role here, especially visceral obesity. Do you have a lot of fat around the middle of your body? If you are male and your waist is greater in circumference than your hips, you have visceral obesity. If you are female and your waist is at least 80% of the circumference of your hips, you have visceral obesity. Visceral obesity causes insulin resistance and plays an important role in developing both impaired fasting glucose and type 2 diabetes.

If you need some help breaking your addiction, please get it.

Simply keep your daily carb consumption very low, which means a maximum of 25 grams daily. Furthermore, eliminate permanently all concentrated or fast-acting carbs and get all your carbs from low-carbohydrate (preferably organic) vegetables.

If you are an addict, admit it. That can be difficult, but you won't cure your addiction without doing it.

Once you think of yourself as an addict, you'll realize that you cannot have treats of fast-acting carbs. Period. For life.

Make no exceptions. If you were trying to quit smoking, you wouldn't allow yourself one cigarette every day, would you? If you were trying to quit a heroin addiction, you wouldn't allow yourself a fix every weekend, would you? Exceptions only keep you addicted. They draw out the process of quitting.

The good news is that, for almost everyone, once you go on a low-carb diet and eliminate all fast-acting carbs from your diet, nearly all your food cravings will soon vanish. Once you break the addiction, you probably won't have cravings like them ever again. (You may, though, experience psychological cravings, but we'll deal with those later, too.)

Remember, following the eating program promoted in this chapter is <u>working with your body</u>. It's eating naturally. It's a diet that promotes a (small!) healthy percentage of body fat as well as overall health and longevity. It's how to work with Mother Nature.

Being addicted to sugar is, like being addicted to dairy products, unnatural. You learned how to be an addict, and you can unlearn how, too.

If given a choice, your body will metabolize sugar rather than fat. It's easier. To improve your percentage of body fat, it's necessary to switch your body from sugar burning to fat burning.

How? Just keep your daily carb intake very low. Yes, doing that may spawn cravings, headaches, and other endurable obstacles *for several days*, but, if you stick with it, they may disappear in 72 hours or less and never return. Whether it takes 2 days or 2 weeks, so what? Freedom isn't free, and that's a small price to break a carb addiction.

Liberty or slow suicide?

If you have never have gone a single day in your adult life without food cravings, you are in for an enduring sense of lightness that will feel much, much better than the temporary taste of anything you can put into your mouth.

Notice what you do when you are feeling full and still crave enjoying continued good tastes. What do you eat? That's right: carbohydrates that turn to simple sugars. There always seems to be room for an extra slice of cake or another pancake with syrup. Notice that, by way of contrast, you don't take, say, a second steak. Since our bodies did not evolve eating lots of carbohydrates, it's not surprising that they have difficulty sending out satiation signals with respect to them.

Similarly, do you ever crave dairy products like ice cream? If so, you are probably addicted to dairy products.

It's simple to test yourself. For ten or fourteen days, simply eliminate whatever you are testing for (whether carbs or grains or dairy products) from what you eat. If as you read this you immediately sense that, for you, that would be difficult to do, it's because, down deep, you already have an inkling that you are an addict.

If you have any thought at all like that, please test yourself. It's simple, but, if you are an addict, you'll find it at least as enlightening as it is difficult. Detailed instructions for testing yourself are readily available.[37] Please do so.

The following is so important that it can be a matter of life and death for some people: *how you feel depends upon the health of your brain, and the health of your brain depends largely upon how you eat* (unless, of course, your have a neurological disease).

Dr. Linus Pauling: "The mind is a manifestation of the structure of the brain itself." Julia Ross: "a healthy, balanced body cannot have chronic mood and weight problems." Joan Mathews Larson, Ph.D.: "A sane and stable mind is possible only with an organically healthy brain."

Yes, (1) it may be uncomfortable to admit that you are an addict, but it's the first step towards freedom. (2) The second step is to eliminate what you are addicted to—and the diet presented in this chapter that is based on healthful, natural fats and proteins will help a lot and enable you to enjoy the benefits of doing so. It may be that temporary amino acid supplementation would also be beneficial in your case.

For additional motivation, just reread the Preface. That's quite a list, isn't it? Many problems such as despair, depression, anxiety, and anger that you think are only emotional problems may be caused by having an unhealthy brain.[38]

Again, (1) if you are having a problem, admit it to yourself. Then (2) put yourself on the natural diet recommended in this chapter and, if necessary, tweak it using suggestions from experts like Ross and Larson in order to tailor it perfectly to your situation. If that does not completely eliminate the problem, following the other steps of The Killing Cravings Method will either eliminate it or reduce it to merely an occasional annoyance.

You now understand in general how to free yourself from cravings and addictions to sugar, carbs and dairy products. (Actually, these are toxins and your body secretes chemicals to soothe itself after you ingest them. What you are really addicted to are those chemical reactions.)

So, what should you eat?

General recommendations may not apply to you. You have individual likes and dislikes. You may have certain food intolerances or allergies. You may be a vegetarian.

You also may have certain other physical conditions that preclude your eating certain kinds of foods. Consult your personal physician (and do some research). For example, consuming foods that contain yeast like baked goods, pickled foods, vinegar, fermented foods, and fermented beverages all can cause problems for people with autoimmune diseases. For example, consuming saturated fats and egg yolks can cause problems for those whose cholesterol ratio is too high.[39]

On the other hand, eating well, which is eating naturally, may be effective treatment for certain physical conditions that plague you. For example, the natural diet recommended in this chapter has proven effective when used to treat type 2 diabetes, sugar cravings and addiction, dairy cravings and addiction, binge eating, mood disorders, obesity, irritable bowel syndrome, acne, allergies, menopause symptons, asthma, inflammation, arthritis, joint pains, epilepsy, and the other conditions and dis-eases listed in the Preface.

Is that really so amazing?

Food is the best medicine. It makes sense that eating the way our bodies evolved to eat is likely to predispose us to being healthy.

If you have freed yourself from cravings for carbs and, similarly, from cravings for dairy products, and are otherwise healthy, what kinds of foods should you eat? It's simple: <u>eat the kinds of foods that are reasonably close to what your successful ancestors actually ate.</u>

Furthermore, as long as they are low carb and, so, won't cause blood sugar spikes (which are not good for you whether or not you happen to be diabetic or prediabetic), civilization has also provided us with an abundance of foods to consider.
Just use the two guidelines concerning proteins and carbs presented earlier in this chapter to select lots of delicious, satisfying foods to eat.

Most meals should be simple and natural such as some fish and a salad or some meat and a vegetable.

However, as long as you stay within the two guidelines and are healthy, you can, if you prefer, occasionally make them complex and unnatural.

It's easy to find lots of low carb recipes in books, on television, and online that yield delicious foods if you want to go to the trouble to prepare them. In the Selected Bibliography list at the end of this book, I've marked with an 'R' books that contain recipes that may work well for you.

Furthermore, and here comes some really good news, if you are healthy and they don't disagree with you, you can try lots of foods that were not available to your successful hunter-gatherer ancestors as long as those foods don't cause blood sugar spikes.[40]

Except for a small amount of berries, that eliminates all modern fruits (including tomatoes) and fruit juices, but there's still a lot of delicious choices left.

For example, you can try many vegetables not already mentioned such as avocado, brussels sprouts, sauerkraut, eggplant, small amounts of onions, and string beans.

You may try almost any kind of meat, fish, fowl, seafood, or organic eggs.

It's best to avoid processed meats such as bologna and other lunch meats, ham, bacon, and sausage. Why? They contain salt and other additives that can cause cravings. If you put yourself on a low salt diet for a couple of weeks, you may be amazed at how much your cravings decrease and how much your interest in eating decreases.

If you are healthy, you may use some (unsalted) butter, cream, and cheeses other than cottage cheese.

Adding sugar is not a good practice. Using any artificial sweetener is problematic (because they may promote blood sugar spikes), but consider experimenting with an occasional serving.

There's nothing necessarily harmful about coffee, tea, seltzer, mineral water, or club soda. There's also sugar-free gum.

If you are not an alcoholic, you may even have a limited amount of alcohol. 'Limited' here means not more than one drink daily for a woman or two drinks daily for a man. (Dark beer, ale, stout, and porter contain considerably more carbs than lighter-colored varieties.)

What about dessert? Try organic berries or ready-to-eat sugar-free Jell-O brand gelatin. (It's especially delicious with a dollop of freshly whipped cream!)

Any self-pity you have about feeling deprived may be more than compensated for by feeling more alert, healthier, lighter, and freer.

Exercise 10

Using foods that you know you'll enjoy eating, write down one day's meals in accordance with the guidelines presented in this chapter. [I've done that work for you in my inexpensive How to Eat Less – Easily!]

Once you have that, you'll have a template you can use frequently. Most people eat mostly the same foods for most of their meals. If you give yourself some variety in at least the chief fat & protein source of the meal you have around dinnertime (for example, steak instead of chicken or sockeye salmon instead of lamb chops), it's not even necessary to vary the salad, vegetable, or, if any, dessert.

WATER

Though it comes last in this chapter, I have not yet mentioned the most important nutrient, namely, water.

When you follow a natural diet, you will almost certainly lose body weight. Why?

You'll be cutting carb consumption. Carbs are stored in our bodies as glycogen, which is a starchy substance used by the body when blood sugar falls too low. Each gram of glycogen is stored with three grams of water. When you cut carb consumption, glycogen will degrade quickly and release the water stored with it. Again, don't confuse losing body weight with losing fat.

It's important to drink plenty of water. It's the primary solvent in your body. It dissolves vitamins, minerals, amino acids, glucose, and other nutrients. It also helps to transport, digest, and absorb nutrients.

Water is a natural diuretic. It flushes out elements like sodium, which is good. With insufficient water consumption, your body will retain water and may look and feel bloated. So it's important to drink plenty of clean water.[41]

How much water should you drink daily?

Again, you are unique. The answer depends upon a variety of factors. Normally, though, it should be at least two quarts. There's no problem drinking three quarts, four quarts, or even more if the weather is hot and humid or you are doing a lot of physical work or exercise.

Also, if you are trying to lose weight, drinking a glass of water shortly before eating a meal works to reduce appetite.

Furthermore, water has a thermogenic effect if it is chilled. In other words, your body has to expend calories to raise the temperature of chilled water. So, drinking plenty of chilled water will actually help you to lose weight.

Incidentally, the idea of a thermogenic effect is one of the reasons the diet promoted in this chapter works so well to reduce body fat. Again, the thermic effect of the different categories of foods is different.

Although the natural eating plan promoted here is not a high protein diet, it is still relatively high in protein in the sense that about one-third of calories consumed come from proteins. One reason that's good is because proteins increase the thermic effect. The thermic effect of foods refers to the calories used by your body to digest and use foods. Proteins can elicit up to a 30% thermic effect![42]

So getting plenty of protein (in addition to using fat instead of sugar as fuel) is also a good idea because of its thermic effect.

OBJECTIONS

Finally, remember that we are operating here in the domain of considered opinion, not knowledge. Since there are a host of variables as well as unknowns, it's wise to be humble.

Of course there are objections that may be raised. Feel free to raise them on my blog.[43] Here are three initial ones. What do you think?

First, you might wonder whether or not eating this way is morally wrong because it involves killing animals. Actually, it does not necessarily involve killing animals if you are willing to get sufficient fats and proteins from eggs, dairy products, and plants. (Another alternative would be to limit killing to killing only seafood – not other mammals.) Furthermore, even if it did necessarily involve killing animals, if this is indeed the only diet that best suits our bodies, foregoing killing would mean that we would deliberately be compromising our health. How could it be right to compromise our health? Self-destruction is good?

Second, everyone could not eat this way without our making massive changes such as reducing the scale and types of farms and ranches, reducing human population, and restoring a lot of the damage that we have done to the earth's ecosystem. Yes, so? It has seemed obvious to me since I was a teenager that there are far too many humans and that we have done enormous damage to our planet. Why not dramatically cut the birth rate and adopt a much more sustainable approach to the environment?[44]

Third, in terms of carb intake, aren't weekly cheat meals beneficial? They are psychologically and, because they encourage the body not to go into starvation mode and slow its metabolic rate (by boosting leptin levels), they may be physiologically beneficial as well. (To begin to learn more about this, use the search bar at http://www.lasting-weight-loss.com/ .)

It's quite simple, though, for you to **test** these ideas for yourself. Just eat this way for a month and observe what happens. What else are you doing that is more important than figuring out how to eat well so that you are as healthy and energetic as possible?[45]

When you develop a way to eat well that works well for you, everything else in your life will become better and more enjoyable.

That's a terrific outcome for the first step, and you'll begin enjoying its benefits within days as soon as you begin doing whatever it takes.

7: Taking Better Control of Your Fitness

Are you willing to improve your fitness seriously by working hard for a total of only **6 to 10 minutes weekly?**

That is exactly what I suggest that you do. This second step of The Killing Cravings Method is to begin doing two fitness sessions each week that consist of a brief warm-up, a 3-to-5 minute work stage, and a brief cool-down. If the warm-ups and cool-downs each take about 3 minutes, which they should, to incorporate sufficient fitness exercise into your life you'll need to spend just *6 to 10 minutes total time doing fitness exercise weekly!*

Obviously, this undermines the "I don't have enough time" excuse. Since doing it will actually boost your energy level, the "I don't have enough energy" excuse also goes out the window.

If, instead of doing brief, intense fitness exercise, you prefer to do longer, less intense fitness exercise, that, too, is an option. I'm referring here to mild fitness exercise such as brisk walking. You may add it on days when you don't do the brief, intense exercising <u>if</u> you want to. Alternatively, if you are willing to spend more time on fitness exercise, you may choose to do no fitness exercise other than mild fitness exercise. It's better than nothing.. This option junks the "I hate intense exercise" excuse.

If you have never been fit, you'll be amazed to discover that you'll get more energy back from fitness (aerobic) exercising than you put into it.

So, with several important "buts" out of your way, let's get started.

If you are a typical Boomer, you don't get enough exercise. You've heard a lot about the benefits of exercise, but that hasn't moved you to do enough.

Exercise is as close to a Fountain of Youth as it's possible to get.

Because there's no association of health experts that doesn't recommend it, you surely already understand that it benefits your health.

Any decent exercise program will increase your cardiovascular efficiency and endurance, improve your flexibility, improve your body composition by promoting fat loss and muscular gains, strengthen and thicken bones and connective tissues, and improve your neuromuscular system.

Sufficient exercise provides dozens and dozens of physiological benefits, including ones related to the discussion in the previous chapter such as reducing your likelihood of suffering a heart attack or stroke, reducing your desire to overeat, reducing insulin resistance, and lowering blood sugar levels.

Perhaps even as important, if you haven't been getting sufficient exercise and begin, you are really going to appreciate its psychological benefits. It not only feels really good, but it will help strengthen your mental outlook and may also have social benefits.

Furthermore, proper progressive exercise is safe. It's also relatively inexpensive and not very time consuming.

However, especially if you are old enough to be a Boomer, please get the blessing of your personal physician before embarking on any exercise program.

Our bodies are moved by our muscles contracting in opposite pairs typically moving tendons that move bones. Your arm will bend when you contract your biceps and it will straighten again when you contract your triceps.

Whenever you move, your muscles use high-energy compounds from glucose or fatty acids to contract. It's convenient to sort exercise into two kinds, namely, <u>fitness</u> or aerobic ("with oxygen") exercise and <u>strength training</u> or anaerobic ("without oxygen") exercise. The metabolic processes involved in fitness exercise derive the required high-energy compounds from small amounts of glucose and large amounts of oxygen, whereas the metabolic processes involved in strength training derive the required high-energy compounds from large amounts of glucose and almost no oxygen.

Fitness exercise is about moving light loads for relatively long durations, while strength training is about moving heavy loads for relatively short durations.

If, as I hope, you want to enjoy optimal benefits from exercise, **it's necessary to do both kinds of physical exercise**. Fitness exercise is the topic of this chapter; strength training is the topic of Chapter 9.[46]

So people are divisible into four categories in terms of exercise. Some do no regular exercise at all. Some only do fitness exercise. Some only do strength training. Some do both fitness and strength training exercise. It's impossible to follow The Killing Cravings Method properly without doing both kinds of exercise.

If you are in one of the first three groups just mentioned, this will require a significant improvement in your regular rituals. I'm going to assist you in improving your exercise habits by making them as simple, easy, and natural as possible. They probably won't require as much time as you think, and the benefits from both kinds of exercise are too important to miss if you are serious about killing cravings and living better.

As long as you are physically normal, **improving your thinking is the key to initiating and sustaining an exercise program.** Use your self-understanding to make it as easy as possible on yourself.

For example, I find strength training fun. I enjoy challenging myself to get stronger. Yes, it's hard work, but it is of short duration and I know from direct experience from many years of doing it that its many benefits are immense. On the other hand, I find prolonged fitness training boring. The Graded Exercise Protocol (abbreviated "GXP") that I present in this chapter, though, is not boring.

Your challenge is to find something that is enjoyable enough for you to keep doing it. There are many options for both kinds of exercise.

Remember that our successful ancestors moved much more than we do. We evolved walking as well as moving and carrying things. At least in North America, most of our lives have become much more sedentary than those of our successful Stone Age ancestors.

Understanding the problem isn't curing it. I show you how to cure it in this chapter and in Chapter 9 with a minimum of physical exertion. Just get yourself doing the minimum regularly and sustain it. That's the purpose of these two chapters.

Warning! You may surprise yourself: you may enjoy moving again so much that you may find yourself regularly doing more than the minimum. (I write 'again' because you almost certainly did a lot of running and jumping around back when you were a kid.)

Exercise is like medicine: too little isn't effective and too much is counterproductive. Your task is to find the right dose, the middle way, that works well for you.

If you do too little, you won't see any lasting improvements and that will predispose you to quit. If you do too much, you may suffer from overtraining, which will predispose you to injuries that may prompt you to quit.

No activity is without risk. Lying on your sofa isn't without risk. While its timing is uncertain, death is certain. There's no birth without death.

In fact, though, not exercising is more dangerous than exercising properly.

Montaigne: "My life has been full of terrible misfortunes, most of which never happened."

There are *three general guidelines* I strongly recommend with respect to fitness exercise that dramatically cut the odds that you'll injure yourself.

<u>First</u>, insist before you begin that your physician do an exercise (stress) electrocardiogram. (This is not the same as a resting or recovery electrocardiogram.) It's not a perfect test; however, it's an extremely effective one in the hands of a well-trained internist or cardiologist.

<u>Second</u>, when exercising, <u>never</u> let your actual heart rate exceed 85% of your predicted maximum heart rate.

<u>Third</u>, <u>always</u> cool-down after fitness exercise; never just stop cold.

With respect to minor injuries, especially if you fail to pay attention to what you are doing, you could strain or sprain something occasionally. If a minor injury occurs, use RICE (rest, ice, compression, elevation) and be patient until it heals.

With respect to overuse injuries, if you follow the guidelines of The Killing Cravings Method, they won't occur.

You could, though, suffer from overtraining – especially if you get very enthusiastic about strength training. Overtraining is a sign that you have lost balance. When in doubt, rest too much rather than too little.

Here are the chief symptoms of overtraining: frequent colds; frequent minor injuries; persistent soreness or stiffness in muscles, joints, or connective tissues; loss of enthusiasm for exercising; inability to relax; difficulty sleeping well; loss of appetite; headaches; and a decrease in performance in your usual work.

Your ability to recover from exercise is limited. Too much exercise can be worse than too little. [I return to this topic in the next chapter.] So please don't overdo exercise.

I recommend either GXP, P.A.C.E. [Progressively Accelerating Cardiopulmonary Exertiion], or interval training twice weekly. I here explain GXP, but, if you understand how to do either P.A.C.E. or interval training properly and prefer it, you may do one of those instead.

GXP is the product of Dr. Robert Otto, Ralph Carpinelli, Ed.D., and Richard Winet, Ph.D.[47] Here's what you'll need:

A heart rate monitor.

Your heart rate numbers.

A fitness exercise machine

Never do GXP without a heart rate monitor. It's impossible to follow the second exercise guideline mentioned on the previous page without one. If you purchase one with a replaceable battery, it will last for many years.[48]

With respect to your heart rate numbers, if you happen to know your actual numbers based on standard exercise testing, use those. If, as is probable, you don't, calculate them. There are different methods to calculate your age predicted heart rate numbers.

The most common method is easy to calculate. (i) Subtract your age from 220. (ii) To calculate your maximum allowable heart rate, take 85% of that number. (iii) To calculate your minimum allowable heart rate, take 80% of that number.[49] For example, if you are 55 years old, the initial number is 165 [220 minus 55]; 85% of 165 is 140 and 80% of 165 is 132. So during the work stage of GXP, continuously monitor your heart rate for the 3 (or

4 or 5) minutes and keep it between 132 and 140 simply by speeding up or slowing down.

Although it can work with other exercise machines, the best exercise machine is a stationary bike, either a traditional upright model (I use a Schwinn Airdyne) or recumbent (reclining) model. You may also use a stair-stepper or a similar machine.

The training program is very simple. GXP has three stages: warm-up, work, and cool-down.

The warm-up stage lasts about three minutes. Simply begin using your machine and gradually increase your pace until your heart rate reaches your 80% (lower) number.

The cool-down stage also lasts about three minutes. Simply decrease your pace until your heart rate gets below 50% of your maximum (higher) number. (If this recovery stage lasts more than about three minutes, you were training too hard for your condition. Don't work quite so hard next time.)

The work stage is simple: just keep your heart rate between your 80% and 85% numbers for the appropriate number of seconds.

To get started, your work stage should last only a few seconds the first time and then, over a number of training sessions, last a bit longer each time until your work stage lasts for three minutes. For example, you might begin with 15 seconds and then increase your time by 15 seconds each session. Your first session work stage will last only 15 seconds, your second session work stage will last 30 second, your third session work stage will last 45 seconds and so on until you reach 180 seconds.

That's it! **Do two sessions weekly until your dotage.**

(You will likely find that GXP is progressive, in other words, as your fitness improves you'll be exercising more intensely.)

If you want to improve your degree of fitness even more, slowly increase the duration of your work stages until they last for 4 or even 5 minutes.

If you want to improve your degree of fitness even more than that, do 3 GXP sessions with 5-minute work stages each week instead of two.

Be careful about doing more than that because, again, your ability to recover from exercise is limited and if you follow The Killing Cravings Method you'll also be doing two strength training sessions weekly.

Nevertheless, you may also want to walk in addition to GXP or you may want to walk instead of doing GXP. After all, we certainly evolved walking. We humans are great walkers. Walking is quintessentially human exercise.

If you already know you'll prefer longer mild fitness exercise to brief more intense fitness exercise like GXP or interval training, what should you do?

Put yourself on a walking program. I have a number of pages at lasting-weight-loss.com that provide specific instructions as well as detailed tips and two beginning programs to choose from.[50]

Exercise 11

Plan your 2 weekly GXP sessions in writing. When will you do them? Where will you do them? What equipment do you need?

(*If* you are also going to walk, add that into your plan. Where are you going to walk? Do you have what you need [for example, walking shoes and a watch]? Be careful not to do too much too quickly. It might be best to wait until you have all 6 steps of The Killing Cravings Method incorporated into your rituals even before adding a walking session weekly.)

If, by the end of your second (or fourth) month, you are eating well and getting sufficient fitness exercise, you may well already find yourself feeling better than you have in years.

You are going to find your life getting better and better as you incorporate the other 4 steps into your daily rituals.

Enjoy the process!

8: Taking Better Control of Your R & R

Pay attention.

Wisdom requires paying attention. If you really want to live better, practice paying better attention. <u>Full focus on the present moment is the key to a full life.</u>

This means living in your thoughts as little as possible. Your thoughts are not your life. The more entangled you are in your thoughts, the less engaged in your life you are. The more you let go of your thoughts, the more your life will flow. Practicing full engagement is the way to more optimal experiences.

This makes sense: since separation is the cause of dissatisfaction and your thoughts are separated from your life, the more you focus on your thoughts the more separated you are from your life.

In addition to developing a daily breathing practice to develop focus [see Chapter 11], the most effective way to get in the habit of doing this is to live in focused bursts of paying attention.

Two chapters ago I recommended adopting a 4X natural eating plan. Usually meals on such a plan will be simpler and shorter. I recommended eating them without distraction.

Is this too complicated or time consuming? Not at all. For example, if you are at work and need to eat a meal, simply sit quietly for a couple of minutes while you enjoy, say, some cold chicken and a salad.

In the previous chapter I recommended exercising for fitness in work stages of just 3 to 5 minutes twice weekly. During those brief but intense stages, I recommended focusing on your heart rate. That is also neither too complicated nor time consuming.

In the following chapter, I recommend exercising for strength twice weekly in brief, intense workouts. Nor is that too complicated or time consuming. As you get stronger, because lapses in concentration can result in injury you'll discover that it's difficult not to pay attention when you are in the gym under relatively heavy iron.

Focused Bursts

Similarly, I recommend working on whatever your Project [see below] is in a focused way. Work intently without interruption for a while and then completely focus on relaxing for a while before another burst of work. This helps to keep the mind unified rather than scattered.

A work burst may last 10 minutes or 4 hours. Individuals differ. Many seem comfortable with work bursts of 60 or 90 minutes followed by a 20 or 30 minute break. Don't focus on work during breaks and don't focus on breaks during work. When you take a break, eat a meal, do a GXP session, go for a walk, or take a nap. If you were to do two work/break sequences twice in the morning and twice in the afternoon, you'd make much more progress on your Project than working distractedly for hours and hours on end.

When you work, focus fully on working. When you relax, focus fully on relaxing. Many people seem to be half working and half relaxing most of the time. They perpetually live in the brown zone. It's foolish to lay bricks while chatting with someone. Instead, get fully into the flow of the work.

Find your most productive time of the day and focus on maximizing your productivity during that time. Though a small minority of people are not morning people, usually the most productive time of the day is the first hour or two after waking up. Go to bed early, get up early, and develop a morning routine that reflects your values.

The "morning pages" exercise is one I recommend that you consider for inclusion in your morning routine.[51] Another is GXP [see the previous chapter] and a third is meditation [see Chapter 11].

It's usually easy to determine your sweet spot during the day: find a way to measure your performance at different times. As a college professor grading papers, exams, or journal entries, I was able to get twice as much done in an hour in the morning as I could get done in an hour in the afternoon or evening. If it took me an hour to grade five papers in the morning, it would take me two hours to grade five papers later in the day.

The psychological key to improving your rest and relaxation (R & R) is to let go of disturbing or distracting thoughts. Relax completely by focusing on relaxing completely.

Never indiscriminately give others the power to interrupt you. Show me someone who answers the phone whenever it rings or responds to email whenever it happens to arrive or answers the door whenever there's an unexpected knock and I'll show you someone who is less than fully productive.

Regularly work to discipline your mind. If you don't, it will incessantly continue to go on thought trains that distract attention from the present moment. Whenever you catch yourself being lost in thought, instantly bring your attention back to the present moment.

Better Sleeping

What should you focus on if, for example, you suffer from racing mind insomnia? Your breathing. What were you told to do as a child in order to fall asleep quickly? Count something. Exactly! Focus on counting your repetitious breaths; furthermore, once you become good at it, a daily breathing practice will help undermine sleep difficulties.

That will not necessarily, however, cure an inability to fall asleep quickly, an inability to stay asleep, or an inability to sleep deeply enough to wake up refreshed. There may be physiological – not psychological – causes to be eliminated.

Occasionally enduring a sleep difficulty is normal and nothing to worry about. Sometimes the causes of such difficulties are apparent and temporary. Did a loved one just die or leave you? Did you just fly across five time zones? Are you ill?

Common physiological, temporary causes of sleep difficulties are indigestion, muscle aches, infections, medications, and food additives. There are also less common ones such as drug withdrawal.

If you are regularly enduring sleep difficulties, there's a lot that you can do.

Do you need to do anything different? Perhaps not. Are you comfortable and alert during the day? Are you able to fall asleep quickly at night? Are you able to sleep through the night? Do you feel refreshed upon awakening?

If not, it's important to establish better sleep rituals. If your personal physician doesn't have any suggestions that work, do some research. Do not fall into the habit of using sleep aids such as over-the-counter sleep medications or, worse, prescription drugs. Instead, try to diagnose the cause or causes of your difficulties and eliminate them.

Begin keeping a written record of your daily rituals so that, when you encounter sleep difficulties, you may be able to use it to identify and test patterns of behavior that might be causing them.

For example, are you eating well? Are you regularly getting the right dose of exercise for you? Have you exercised within 3 hours of retiring for the night? Have you finished most of your daily water intake by late afternoon? Have you eliminated caffeine from all sources? Do you use any supplements (like phosphatidylserine [PS]) that may be interfering with normal sleep habits?

Is your bedroom dark enough? Is its temperature conducive for sleep? Do you have a good mattress? If you sleep with someone, might that person be disturbing your sleep?

Is your pre-sleep ritual conducive for sleep? Minimize agitations. Do not listen to or watch the news in the 4 hours before retiring. Do not associate with people who have agitated minds in the hours before retiring. Avoid alcohol, tobacco, and nonprescription drugs in the evenings.

A warm, relaxing bath or a massage before bed can help. The best pre-sleep ritual is meditation.

Whether or not you meditate, another good one is progressive relaxation. There are different ways to do it; the general method is to flex a muscle group hard for 6 seconds, completely relax it, and move on to the next group. Work up from your toes to your feet and then on to your calves, shins, hamstrings, thighs, buttocks, abdomen, chest, upper back, hands, forearms (front and back), biceps, triceps, shoulders, and neck.

Avoid sleeping on your back or stomach. Sleep on your side with your thighs perpendicular to your spine with a small pillow between your knees (to ease the strain on your lower back) and another pillow supporting your neck (to keep your upper spine straight). Keep your arms down rather than over your head, which will prevent shoulder problems. To switch sides, just swing your knees up and roll over. If you don't already sleep this way, it's easy to train yourself to do it automatically.

If you are unable to sleep well and are unable to help yourself, get some professional help. Unknown to you, you may be suffering from sleep apnea, narcolepsy, somnambulism, or bruxism (grinding your teeth at night). You may need help to deal with nightmares or night terrors. There are professionals who may be able to help you. Discuss with your physician the possibility of visiting a sleep lab.

Don't settle for living with sleep difficulties. Think of it this way: one of the most effective tortures is simply to deprive someone of sleep. It's nearly impossible to live well without being able to sleep well.

Exercise 12

Write down a pre-sleep ritual that may work well for you. Include what time you'll be going to bed and when you'll regularly be arising. If you plan well and stick to your plan, you may never again need to use an alarm clock. (I never do.)

Better Vacationing

Excellent R & R is not just about sleeping well; it's also about vacationing well.

Personally, I think of daily meditation sessions as short daily vacations. They are as much a break of routine as taking trips sightseeing, camping, or visiting other places or people.

Our English word 'vacation' comes from an old French word that was derived from the Latin word that meant "make empty." So, at least etymologically, vacationing well means making empty well. Making what empty? Vacating what?

The mind.

Nothing is better for stress relief than emptying the mind of thoughts.

(Thinking about vacationing well can also be helpful when we consider how best to live every day.)

There are two important mistakes about vacationing.

The *first mistake* is based on the truth that **nothing abides**. Reality is in ceaseless flux.

What I think of as Bradford's Law of Conditioned Life follows from this most fundamental truth. Where 'G' denotes the satisfaction that comes from gaining whatever is desired and 'L' denotes the dissatisfaction that comes from losing whatever is desired, $G + L = 0$. There are no permanent gains. Our elation when we gain something we want is always balanced by our sadness when we lose it.

For example, the temporary high of falling in love is always balanced by the suffering caused by its end.[52] We like to pretend to ourselves that love affairs are endless, but the reality is that every relationship ends.

If so, it's a major mistake when going on vacation to go intending to gain something you want. The purpose of going on vacation should not be to gain anything. Lasting gains are impossible, and the benefits of temporary gains are always balanced by their costs.

(Similarly, it's a major mistake when going through a day to make gaining something your major priority.)

The *second mistake* is in trying to leave our work behind.

Distinguish 'work' from 'job.' It is not necessary to have a job to live well, but it is necessary to work to live well. Your work is what you choose to do. It's what your life is about, your Project or self-identified purpose or direction (whatever that may be). It's what you do whenever you have the leisure and money to do whatever you want. Your work is what you do and, so, it's the center of your personal identity. It is impossible not to be who you are.

Therefore, it's senseless to try to be who you are not.

Instead of trying to get away from your work by going on vacation, your vacation should be devoted to your work. **Work is play.** (If your work is not play for you, either you are not yet good at it or you are doing the wrong work for you.)

For example, I am a philosopher. My work is to become wise. I intend to master life and to show others how to master life. I've committed myself wholeheartedly to doing whatever it takes. My thoughts are my biggest obstacle to success. So my most important work is freeing myself from bondage to my own thoughts.

(This work is not just about me. I do it for others. Why? If successful, my life will automatically become a model for others. The great sequence is: learn, do, then show or teach others. To free myself from my thoughts is to free myself from egocentricity, which is moving from selfishness to selflessness. Again, it is selfless sages who are the greatest lovers. For more on this, see my <u>Love and Respect</u>.)

What, then, would be a great vacation for me? It's to spend a week on a zen retreat. For the most part, they are conducted in silence and involve a minimum of ten hours daily of formal meditation. Demanding? Yes. Painful? Yes. Liberating? Well, the goal is emptying the mind of all thoughts. Since that's the purpose of going on vacation, at least for me a zen retreat is a great vacation.

If you think of vacations as a break from drudgery, then the job you are fleeing is not your work. If that's the case, ask yourself whether or not there is some way to make your job your work. If you do, then you'd be bringing your values and your daily life into much better alignment.

You might wonder whether or not it is possible to vacation well without a purpose (Project). The answer is, "No." Since lacking a purpose means being pointless, without a purpose everything is pointless.

You might not have a purpose and wonder how to get one. Look for it! Do you think it will magically knock you on the head as you are drinking beer watching television?

You might wonder how to look for your purpose. Try this: get up early enough in the morning to have two hours of quiet by yourself. Sit down with a pen and a blank piece of paper. Think about possibilities and jot down ideas. Do that every morning for as long as it takes. When you find it, begin to make all your decisions about what to do on the basis of whether or not the proposed actions might get you closer to your purpose. In other words, set your goals that foster your Project in writing and use instrumental reason to work towards them.

Avoid living a life focused on achieving goals. Though it initially seems counter-intuitive, sages lead lives detaching from achieving goals (which is their Project). [For more on this, see my Mastery in 7 Steps.]

Here is another hint in addition to ones I've dropped before: might your purpose really be a loss rather than a gain?

Exercise 13

Write down your Project. Try to boil it down to just one sentence.

Do the other goals that you have been writing down in the course of this book serve your Purpose? If not, revise them until they do.

Here's a final suggestion about R & R: **stop hurrying**. Surely you don't think of hurrying through it as having a good vacation. A good vacation should not involve hurrying.

Neither should your everyday life.

Sadly, the hurry syndrome is ubiquitous. In fact, you may be so accustomed to speeding through life that you don't even notice it, and, if you do happen to notice it, the habit of hurrying may have so much momentum in your life that it seems impossible to slow it down even just a little.

Reforming our deeply engrained rituals is never easy.

There's no substitute for using some time during your morning ritual to plan your daily activities and to resolve not to rush through them.

Do you want to rush through a meal? Do you want to rush though a strength training session? Do you want to rush through a conversation with a friend? Do you want to rush though making love or enjoying a sunrise or gazing on a seascape?

Henry David Thoreau: "I have no time to be in a hurry."

Make your work your play, and don't rush through it.

9: Taking Better Control of Your Strength

The best is yet to come.

If you have spent at least a month implementing each of the previous 3 steps of the Killing Cravings Method, congratulations! You should feel very good about your progress.

Exercise 14

Take a few moments to recall in as much detail as possible exactly how you felt three (or six) months ago. Remember your struggle to gain control of your eating. It wasn't easy! The benefits, though, of how you feel, how much your energy level has increased, and, perhaps, how your health has begun to improve are probably already significant and will become even more important in the future. Whatever your initial results, take a few moments to write them down.

As the old saying goes, the shortest pencil is better than the longest memory.

Was doing some brief but intense fitness exercise twice weekly a struggle? Even if it was, you have already begun to feel much better physically, haven't you? If it wasn't because you were already doing sufficient fitness exercise, you have at least gained confidence that your program really has been working for you. Jot down your initial results.

Have you intensified and regularized your rituals with respect to rest and relaxation? If so, there's been an obvious improvement in how you feel. They will begin to serve you even better as you initiate strength training.

Furthermore, there's more stress reduction training to come (Chapter 11). Write down your initial results.

For real: it will keep getting better. Persist.

The purpose of this chapter is to encourage you to **do serious strength training twice weekly.** That's the 4th step of The Killing Cravings Method.

It's beyond the scope of this chapter to explain in detail how to do that. For details on how to do the minimum, see my <u>Weight Lifting</u>. Here I offer you the next best encouragement by telling you exactly how to get any questions you may have answered easily.

What is strength training and why does it matter?

Let's start with what it's not: it's neither bodybuilding nor weightlifting.

Bodybuilders use resistance training in an effort to sculpt their bodies to make them more aesthetically pleasing. Bodybuilders compete aesthetically. You probably will lose body fat and gain muscle, but gaining a more beautiful body is not the goal here. It is, possibly, a secondary benefit.

Whether it's power lifting or Olympic lifting, weight lifting is all about lifting the most amount of weight doing single repetitions in various ways. It's a competitive sport. Weightlifters use resistance training to do better at weightlifting contests. Although you will get somewhat stronger, you never have to enter any such contests or train for them.

While there is a correlation between strength and muscle mass, how strong you are is <u>not</u> only a function of the cross-sectional size of your major muscle groups; it's also a function of other physiological factors such as the strength of your tendons and how much leverage you happen to have (in terms of the length of certain bones).

This leads to an important point: again, <u>you are unique</u>. Nobody has your genes. Because of genetic differences, there is a wide variation in outcomes from strength training. Even using similar eating programs, similar R & R rituals, and similar strength training protocols, some people will gain considerable muscle mass, some people will gain considerable strength, some people will gain both considerable strength and muscle mass, some people will gain considerable muscle mass but not considerable strength, some people will gain considerable strength but not considerable muscle mass, and some people will gain only some muscle mass or strength.

If you are a man, you probably would like additional strength and muscle mass.

If you are a woman, you probably would like additional strength (especially upper-body strength) but you probably do not want additional muscle mass. Don't worry: because of the hormonal differences between the sexes, unless you (foolishly!) take anabolic steroids, which are like artificial testosterone, although you may become more shapely as well as stronger, you are not likely to gain much muscle mass.

So, everyone who does strength training properly will become at least somewhat stronger (and some men will also gain considerable muscle mass). However, getting stronger may not matter that much to you and you may not want to gain considerable strength and muscle mass even if that's a possibility for you. So why do any strength training?

Even if you never develop much more strength or muscle mass, strength training has numerous, important benefits. Even setting aside potential social benefits that come from becoming more disciplined, attractive, and confident, what are the mental and physical benefits of training properly for improved strength?

Though immeasurable, the **psychological benefits** are very valuable. For some people, they are simply astounding.

Since, again, the future I unknown ands unknowable, we live in uncertainty about what will happen.

Those who enjoy a positive attitude about life have an important advantage over those who don't. *Doing strength training regularly is one of the best tools available for sustaining a positive attitude.* If you have never done strength training and doubt that (as you should), follow the program presented here and simply pay attention to how your everyday attitude improves in the coming months.

The reason that proper strength training will make you feel better is simple: it's healthful. The healthier you are, the easier it is to enjoy being in a good mood.

There's another important mental benefit that is infrequently mentioned: it predisposes you to handle (physical) pain better. That, in turn, predisposes you to handle suffering better.

At least for chronic pain, researchers have discovered little or no relationship between physical damage that is objectively assessed (physical pathology) and reduced functioning, disability, or the amount of experienced (felt, sensed) pain reported. What matters most is how willing someone is to experience pain and that person's ability to act in a valued direction while experiencing it.

If you have been an athlete, you probably know this from direct experience. You probably have even guessed it if you simply watch athletes; indeed, learning it is one of the ways that great athletes can inspire the rest of us.

Done properly, strength training is very safe. It's certainly safer than the only alternative, namely, not doing any strength training and thereby ensuring that you will endure increasing weakness as you age. Do you really want to be unable to open a window in a heat wave when you get old?

However, it does involve pain. If you have been sedentary for years and began the GXP program presented in Chapter 7, you probably experienced a small amount of pain, perhaps onset muscular soreness during exercise (OMS) or delayed onset muscular soreness a day or two after exercise (DOMS).

Expect the same with strength training. Of course it can be briefly agonizing to lift a (relatively) heavy weight, and, if you go past what you are accustomed to doing, you probably will feel some DOMS as well as OMS. That's normal.

I'm not here talking about sustaining what would ordinarily be thought of as injuries. When pain is a stop signal, as before, use RICE and be patient; don't train for a while.

The normal pain associated with strength training, though, is not a stop signal. It comes from micro-injuries (see below). As long as you don't do too much too quickly, simply think of that kind of pain as a mark of progress. While any physically normal person can bench press a pair of pencils, not many can bench press a pair of 150 pound dumbbells – and those who are able to do that paid the price to be able to do that.

Be willing to push yourself; allow yourself to experience OMS. If you don't during a workout, you won't enjoy the benefits of strength training.

Expect DOMS, too. If you train progressively, DOMS won't slow you down at all. In fact, if I don't feel any DOMS after a day or two, I'm disappointed. I think I must have failed to work hard enough. (Because of adaptability, the more years you train, the less DOMS you may experience.)

Don't want to do GXP today even though it's scheduled? Remind yourself of all those people who are crippled and otherwise physically unable to do intensive fitness training today who would love to be able to do it today. Do the same thing if you are hesitating about a strength training workout.

The truth is that life is sometimes painful. Pain is inevitable. Unlike suffering, which is optional, pain happens. The purpose of pain is to help us survive. As long as the pain from strength training isn't a stop sign, which it almost never is if you use proper exercise technique and progressive resistance, you will become stronger only by being willing to accept it and keep training.

Assuming that pain is not a stop sign, there are two important lessons: (1) always be willing to experience either pain or suffering and (2) always be ready to refuse to let either pain or suffering stop you from doing what you decide to do.

For example, I sometimes hesitate before doing a work set of deadlifts, especially when they are personal bests. They are difficult, painful, and seem to require all my effort. When I think about how the next rep will feel, I can get so entangled in my imaginings that I actually stop myself, either by quitting training for that workout or failing even to break the barbell off the floor. When, though, I ignore my thoughts and just step up to the bar to do my next regularly scheduled set, I usually am able to do it. Then I feel really good about how I failed to let the edge of my previous comfort zone stop me.

In other words, this mental benefit is the extraordinarily valuable benefit of **practicing ignoring your thoughts**. Thoughts are not real; they are only thoughts. A feeling of pain is itself a thought. As long as you notice it and decide that it's not a stop sign, let it go and focus on doing what you have decided to do.

The same goes for emotions like fear. I sometimes fear heavy single deadlifts. (Don't worry: beginning or intermediate trainees will have no such fear because they should never do fewer than 5 repetitions.) I have sometimes felt in the middle of a repetition as though my back would break!

Since my technique is perfect and I train progressively, it never has. In fact, I don't recall *ever* having been injured at all doing deadlifts. I've recently done deadlifts using well over 400 lbs. and, while that's not much for power lifters, it's not bad for an ex-hockey player in his mid-60's who'd just like to be as healthy as possible.

Furthermore, emotions always involve a central delusion.[53] At their heart, all positive emotions involve the thought "this is good for me" and all negative emotions involve the thought "this is bad for me." Those evaluations are nothing but thoughts! They are nothing but egocentric evaluations. Notice them, refuse to get entangled in them by letting them go, and get back to focusing fully on doing what you decided to do.

To return to the point about microscopic injuries: you don't get stronger in the gym. Done properly, what you do in the gym actually tears down muscles and that process continues for many hours after your workout. With proper nutrition and proper R & R, the next day or two your muscles will build themselves up so that they become stronger in response to the overload stimulus you gave them.

So, becoming stronger is a matter of tearing down and building up. If you foolishly thought that you would become stronger while training and, so, tried training for hours every day for days on end, you would actually wind up weaker than before you began. Proper nutrition [Chapter 6] and proper rest & relaxation [Chapter 8] are as important for strength training success as proper training in the gym.

Furthermore, again, your ability to recover from exercise of both kinds is limited. This explains the recommendation to do only brief fitness training sessions twice (or, at most, three times) weekly [Chapter 7]. Similarly, as long as you are doing intense fitness training twice weekly as well as strength training, if possible minimize other physical activities at least until you are certain that they won't cause overtraining.

How frequently should you do strength training? Beginners who are using only the lightest weights can get away with working out three times weekly. Advanced trainees may only train once every 10 or 14 days. For most people, doing strength training twice weekly works best.

However, do not rely on some arbitrary schedule: "listen" to your body. Here's the rule: <u>wait at least 24 hours after all DOMS has disappeared before training again</u>. Waiting 24, 48, or even 72 hours more is fine. This will ensure systemic as well as localized recovery.

Notice the 'all.' If DOMS was stimulated by a whole body routine, which is what all beginners should be using, you'll likely find that DOMS disappears at different rates for different muscle groups. Wait until DOMS has disappeared from <u>all</u> muscle groups before starting the 24 hour clock ticking before your next workout. When in doubt, wait another day before training again.

It's also important to factor in *adpatability*. In a few weeks of using a single strength training routine your body will adapt to it. So every two or three months, take a whole week's rest from strength training and then begin a new routine. Change the exercises or the order of the exercises or the set & repetition combinations you are using.

What if you prefer to exercise on, say, only Mondays and Thursdays? If you want to do GXP and strength training on the same day, that's fine. However, it's best to separate the two sessions by at least 6 hours. If that's impossible, do the GXP after the strength training.

If you want additional exercise in addition to 2X weekly fitness training and 2X weekly strength training, please limit it to brisk walking. Don't exceed 3 miles in 45 minutes and 2 miles in 30 minutes would be better in the beginning. Be careful about doing it more than once weekly in addition to your other workouts.

(Depending upon your physical condition, it can take 20 or 25 minutes before your body begins to burn fat rather than carbs. So, if you are adding brisk walking for fat burning, it should last more than about 25 minutes. More important for improving your body composition is proper nutrition, which includes usually lim-limiting carb intake to 25 grams or fewer daily.)

Consider, too, the **physical benefits** of strength training.

Bone remodeling is a continuous process. Without sufficient weight-bearing exercise, in other words, without using your body weight to stress your skeleton, your bones will weaken by leaching calcium and other minerals and, so, becoming more brittle. Some fitness exercises such as swimming and stationary bicycling are not weight-bearing exercises. Improving bone density is a sufficient reason to do strength training, weight-bearing fitness exercise, or impact exercise. If you do strength training, you don't have to worry about doing weight-bearing fitness exercise or doing impact exercise, which is unnecessarily dangerous. Either use your bones or decrease your ability to use them.

Improved tendon strength is another benefit of strength training.

Perhaps the most important reasons to do strength training exercise relate to your muscles.

For example, even if strength training does not increase your muscle mass, it will still reduce insulin resistance. The greater your muscle mass, the less insulin your body will need, and, since insulin is the chief fat storing hormone, less insulin in your bloodstream means less fat stored and, so, better body composition.

Again, since muscle is much more metabolically active than fat, increased muscle mass will enable you to burn additional calories 24 hours a day.

However, please don't use the fact that you are doing regular fitness exercise or strength training to increase the amount of carbs you consume daily. Many people rationalize increased carb consumption that way and prevent themselves from lowering their percentage of body fat. Unless you are a professional or world-class athlete who spends hours training every day, think of exercise only as a weight loss supplement to the kind of di-dietary plan advocated in Chapter 6.

Strength training has additional health benefits. For example, if you have a genetic tendency to become diabetic or if you are either prediabetic or diabetic, it is extremely beneficial. Insulin helps your body either burn blood glucose or, if there's an ample supply in your bloodstream, store it. The energy from glucose is mainly stored as glycogen, which is a polysaccharide, in the liver or in the muscles or as fat (triglycerides) in fat cells. Typically there's twice as much glycogen stored in muscles as in the liver.

When your body needs quick energy, it uses glucose. Glycogen is used for storing energy short term, and fat is used for storing energy long term. When the short term energy stores are full, your body will store the excess energy as fat.

You want to keep blood glucose levels normally low. The greater your muscle mass, the greater your body's capacity for taking up blood glucose and storing it as glycogen. How do your muscles then deplete the glycogen they store? Mainly through being used or exercised.

So strength training is doubly important: it not only usually increases your muscle mass, but also it allows your muscles to eliminate stored glycogen.

Strength training lowers blood glucose levels both during exercise and for many hours afterwards.

This also helps to explain why it's good to keep dietary carbs low. Carbs are broken down to produce sugars, mostly glucose. Glucose is exactly what people susceptible to diabetes cannot handle, and high blood glucose levels (particularly after meals) are not good for anyone.

The whole exercise program recommended here consists of brief, but intense, workouts doing both fitness and strength training. The benefits of the whole program are greater than the sum of the benefits of its parts. Why? Activity breeds activity; inactivity breeds inactivity.

Fitness and strength lead to more fitness and strength, while obesity leads to further obesity and sedentary living leads to more sedentary living.

Since we are creatures of habit, it's important to establish good habits. It's not easy to establish good habits, but they are much easier to live with than the only alternative.

Frequent strenuous exercise significantly reduces your chances of suffering heart attacks, strokes, or blood vessel obstructions.

Long-term strenuous exercise lowers both your resting heart rate and blood pressure, thus also lowering your risk of cardiovascular events.

Prolonged strenuous exercise can lower blood sugar levels.

(Still, since brief strenuous exercise can raise blood sugar levels as well as blood pressure, these are two specific reasons to get medical clearance before starting either strenuous fitness training or strength training.)

The key to enjoying these benefits is to *train progressively*. Keep doing slightly more or better at each workout. Ensure that each workout is slightly more challenging than the last workout.

Are you convinced? I hope so and that you are eager to learn how get the most benefits from strength training.

Here are the most important guidelines: **Never do dangerous exercises, learn and always use proper exercise technique, start with very light resistance, and proceed progressively.**

Although it's possible to find some excellent free videos on YouTube demonstrating perfect exercise technique, be skeptical about many sources of strength training advice. Much of it is dangerous or incomplete. Much of the rest of it is applicable primarily only to either bodybuilders or weightlifters.

Fortunately, there is one paperback available that provides detailed guidelines that are almost nearly always correct about which exercises to use, how to perform them, and how to set up your own routines. It's Stuart McRobert's Build Muscle Lose Fat Look Great.[54]

Let me anticipate some questions you may have and where to find answers to them. Even if you don't have a copy of McRobert's book, I provide lots of answers that are freely available in the strength training sections of my free website at: http://www.lasting-weight-loss.com/. To save space and increase clarity here, permit me to refer to the relevant pages of this site by only their html designations below. For example, 'strength-training' means 'http://www.lasting-weight-loss.com/strength-training.html' . (Usually, McRobert provides more detailed answers in his book.)

Which exercises are too dangerous? Answer: unless you are an advanced trainee, only use the exercises listed in and described in McRobert's book.

How should I learn perfect exercise technique? Study Part 2 of McRobert's book.

Where should I train? See Part 1 of McRobert's book.

How should I begin? See my 'strength_training'.

How can I do strength training safely? See my 'exercising'.

How can I quickly learn strength training terminology? See my 'strength-training'.

How should I warm-up for strength training? See my 'weight-lifting-tips'.

Should I use a full range of motion? See my 'weight_lifting_tips'.

How should I eat before, during, and after strength training workouts to maximize their benefits? See my 'protein-shakes'.

What are the best exercises to use? See my 'weightlifting-exercises'.

How can I determine what is the best number of repetitions for me to use? There is a way to test your different muscle groups, but you should have been training regularly for at least a year before doing the tests.[55] If you are a beginner, just generally stay between 5 and 20 reps.

What about improving the stability and function of my midsection? See my 'core-strength-exercises'. 'core-exercise', and 'core_exercises'.

What would be a good set of routines for the first year of strength training? See my 'weight-lifting'.

What would be some good routines for intermediate trainees? See my 'weight_lifting'.

What should I do if I encounter obstacles? See my 'obstacles'.

Beverly Sills: "There are no shortcuts to any place worth going."

Does it seem that this step is anything except simple?

It's true that there's a lot to learn if you want to do strength training well. Personally, I think of it as being like learning about a hobby. Hobbies are fun. If they are too simple, if they don't engage our minds, they can become boring.

On the other hand, the workouts themselves are simple. Once you understand how to set up routines that work well for you, the focus shifts to execution.

Since deadlifts, squats, and their variations are the best exercises, it's a good idea to begin every workout, when you are freshest, doing either deadlifts or squats. Try alternating them: start a workout doing deadlifts and start the next workout doing squats and continue that sequence.

Exercise 15

Decide which exercises you will do for your two strength training workouts your first week. Which days will you do them? Where will you do them? How long will you rest between sets? How will you warm-up before training? Which stretches will you use after training?

The first week just do one set of each exercise. The second week do two sets of each exercise. The third week do three sets of each exercise.

Keep the rest time between sets consistent. It may be any time from between 5 to 180 seconds. Feel free to start with a common 60 seconds between sets; however, experiment as the months go by and judge by your results.

Use a whole-body routine each time and alternate routines by basing one each week on (one kind of) deadlifts and the other on (one kind of) squats.

This won't be as difficult as you may initially imagine. It's not complicated. Here are two examples.

Workout A: back squats, bench presses, pulldowns, dumbbell shrugs, and crunches. Workout B: deadlift partials in a power rack, back raises, dumbbell presses, dips, and curls.

Workout B: box squats, back extensions, incline barbell presses, side bends, dumbbell curls, twisting crunches, neck work. Workout B: sumo deadlifts, dips, chins, Arnold presses, gripper work, finger extensions.

Use your alternating A/B workouts for seven (or eleven) weeks, take one week off from any strength training, and then start another eight (or twelve) week program. (There's a first year's worth of programs on my website.)

The basic strength-training exercises are deadlifts, squats, presses, rows, dips, and chins (or pull-downs). Since there are plenty of variations of them and they may be combined in seemingly endless different ways, there's no need ever to get bored.

[Again, see my <u>Weight Lifting</u> for an excellent routine template that requires less than 10 minutes once weekly.]

However, doing a routine really is simple. If you focus on practicing briefly once (or twice) weekly, you'll really be pleased that you did.

Whatever they are, find a way to let go of all your excuses. For example, if you don't have access to resistance training equipment, use a book such as Laura and Clark's <u>You Are Your Own Gym</u> to do strength training without weights or machines. Drop your excuses; train hard but briefly once or twice a week.

10: Taking Better Control of Your Encounters

Once upon a time I had a girlfriend who told me that, when she was in elementary school, she deliberately and regularly practiced befriending kids who were not very popular. She said that's the way her parents raised her.

I thought, "Wow!" I don't recall that I was raised like that; if my parents tried, they failed.

It took me over half a century to realize, even in theory, that, if you want better relationships, **focusing on the other person** is always better than being ego-centric.

My tendency was always to be intensely thoughtful only in the sense that my priority was straightening out my own conceptual thinking. The natural result was that I became very attached to my own thoughts. Though I was always willing to re-examine them, I defended them with such vigor that I often seemed to others intellectually forceful and arrogant.

I tended to relate to others as if they were ideas rather than people. I look back on the first time I fell in love as falling in love with the idea of being in love! I understood my girlfriend as if she were a character in a novel.

I failed to be intensely thoughtful in the sense that I failed to make my priority promoting what would be good for the other person. I was always in my own way in the sense that my encounters (interpersonal relationships) were always filtered through my own thoughts.

Jack Parr: "Looking back, my life seems like one long obstacle race, with me as its chief obstacle."

I became so good at conceptualizing that, eventually, except for an occasional colleague, nobody debated with me anymore. I failed to make it easy for others to relate well to me.

In one way I was a typical male: my concern was wholly with the message. I was blind to the meta-message.

I hope that you weren't as foolish as I was. If you were, I hope that you have let that approach go.

Eventually, about 20 years ago, I became interested in business. That forced me to change my orientation toward others, and I began to read book after book and took course after course on how to succeed in business.

I quickly learned that, "People don't care how much you know until they know how much you care." Since I had been proceeding on the opposite assumption, no wonder many of my encounters had been less than wholly satisfactory. Instead of focusing on others, I had been focusing on improving my own understanding. I assumed that, once others understood how good my intellect was, they'd be attracted to me. Naturally, I was never hesitant to tell them how good it was – with predictable results.

It now seems obvious to me that people really will do business with you if they know, like, and trust you. If worldly success interests you, please understand that it's more important to be likable than it is to be great at theorizing.

The thesis of this chapter is simple: **If you want to have better encounters, take the focus off yourself and focus instead on promoting what is good for others without being at all concerned about what you might gain by doing so.**

That may be, for you, obvious. For me, it was far from obvious; it was a real struggle to learn it.

Once it sunk in, many puzzling occurrences suddenly made sense to me. In the world I lived in, likability was irrelevant. In the everyday world most people live in, likability is extremely important.

Exercise 16

Recall important encounters you've had. Think of ones in which you attempted to gain something from someone else. How did they turn out? Have there ever been any in which you attempted only to give something to someone else? How did they turn out?

Even understanding this, though, is insufficient. It's necessary to practice it regularly.

Let's examine both parts of the thesis of this chapter: first, the idea of focusing on yourself and, second, the idea of promoting what is best for others without thinking of yourself.

First, examining the idea of self undermines egocentricity.

WARNING: Because the material is difficult and this presentation is concentrated, the next two pages may be initially difficult to understand. However, if you work through the material slowly, you'll not only find it interesting but very valuable.

Start with a distinction. A "monadic" quality is had by one individual. For example, a curtain is blue or that rock is hard. A "relational" quality is had by two or more individuals. For example, the door is to the left of the window or Betty is sitting between Al and Charley.

Especially in the west, many people think of themselves as they think of all individuals, namely, as if they were pin cushions stuck full of pins. The pins stand for qualities (properties, attributes, characteristics, features).

The tendency in western thinking is to understand

the qualities that individuals have as monadic qualities. Westerners think or say of someone that he is, for example, honest or lazy or kind or thrifty. The fundamental presupposition is that there is this real thing, this particular individual, separated from everything else and correctly describable in terms of some unique set of monadic qualities.

The tendency in eastern thinking is to understand the qualities that individuals have as relational qualities. Instead of thinking of people as separated units, easterners think of individuals as if they were embedded in a specific context, inseparably related to the whole. The fundamental presupposition is that it is better to describe someone relationally rather than nonrelationally. For example, so-and-so is the daughter of that couple, the mother of that child, the employee of that company, and so on. Personal qualities like honesty, laziness, kindness, or thriftiness are nothing but similarities (identities, commonalities) shared with others rather than differences separating individuals.

On this issue, the eastern view is better. If you are inclined to disagree, ask yourself a simple question: **What is the pin cushion?** When you strip away all the pins, what is left? What is the surd or substratum that remains?

Since it has no qualities, it can't be anything!

As great philosophers like Gotama, Nagarjuna, and Hume have argued, there is no separate object that is an individual. If this underlying pin cushion is thought of as a separate self, then there are no separate selves. To remove all the ways an individual relates to everything else is to remove the individual.

This goes for us humans as well as for rocks, non-human animals, lakes, and clouds. Individuals are not separate selves. It's impossible even to think of what that would be. Instead of being entities separate from and in addition to their qualities, individuals are nothing but clusters of qualities.

It's even possible to prove this to yourself about yourself. How? By direct experience [See Chapter 11].

As this relational style of thinking about individuals becomes more and more familiar, the notion of egocentricity begins to dissolve. Adopting the eastern view intellectually helps to prepare the mind for a thorough awakening.

What if there really is no "you" inside? Who is reading these words? Who is thinking?[56]

Though for you it may be initially very uncomfortable and disconcerting even to think for a moment that you may not be a separate self, you may come to find it very liberating. Why? You are not stuck forevermore being you. Furthermore, you are not necessarily isolated, separate, and lonely.

Fundamentally, liberation from bondage to the ego, freedom from ego delusion, is possible. Realizing that liberation in practice is precisely why the lives of sages flow rather than repeatedly getting stuck.

Again, this material is both difficult and very important.

Once you drop all the storytelling about yourself, you will begin to realize how much energy you have been expending creating and sustaining the myth that you are a separate self. When you think about episodes in your life, isn't your tendency to make yourself into the hero of the story? Aren't others often attempting to mess up your life and only succeed in doing so when you weaken? Aren't you in a kind of constant battle with the unrelenting forces of evil trying to undermine you? Aren't you constantly vigilant about propping yourself up, about keeping the story going?

All that storytelling is unnecessary. That's what sages have realized that the rest of us haven't. Letting go of the incessant narration about ourselves is liberating.

We are free from the heavy burden of having to sustain our identities from one moment to the next.

Even if you adopt the thought that it's false that you are a separate self, that's not the same as realizing it. It's only thinking something. It's just another thought. Realizing it requires letting go of it, directly experiencing thoughts without a thinker. That is a simple idea, but, in practice, it's very difficult to do.

Ultimately, realization dissolves the self/other distinction. Once you realize that you are empty of a separate self, you realize that there is no separation between you and everything else. The more you incorporate this insight into your daily life, the more dissatisfaction evaporates. Why? Again, since dissatisfaction is caused by separation, the less separation there is, the less dissatisfaction there is.

John Daido Loori: "Realizing that you do not exist separately from everything else, you realize responsibility: you are responsible for everything you experience . . . That understanding changes your way of relating to the world . . . There is nowhere to run to, nothing to run from . . ."

Second, in a relative sense, it's false that you are others. You are different from everything else. However, in an absolute sense, since you are empty of a separate self, you are others. You are everything else.

Therefore, in an absolute sense, whenever you promote what is good for others, you are promoting what is good for yourself. Since there's no distinction between the two, what is good for one is also good for the other.

Dogen: "Beneficial action is an act of oneness, benefitting self and others together. . . "

Is this really so very different from what happens frequently in everyday life? We choose what really matters to us and, so, what we identify with. We create ourselves, our identities. We choose our identifications.

For example, a mother may choose to identify with her child. The mother's perspective is that what is good for this child is good for me. The life of that child may be more important to her than her own life. How could the child be a more important part of the mother's self than that? It's impossible to understand the mother without understanding her in relation to her child.

Please wonder about this analysis and about objections to it.

Even if it's impossible to know what to do [recall the argument in Chapter 4], how can one promote what is good for one's friend or beloved (the other)?

It does follow that it impossible to know how to promote what is good for another. Many of life's most agonizing moments come from realizing this truth. You may intensely want your child to stop doing drugs, or your friend to stop engaging in promiscuous sex, or your father to exercise, but you may also be acutely aware that you are ignorant about how to bring about those results.

Even if you don't know how to promote what is good for another, it doesn't follow that you must fail to promote what is good for the other. You could try various experimental approaches and, if you are skillful enough or lucky enough, one might actually work.

Ed Foreman: "You can never tell what type of impact you may make on another's life by your actions or lack of action. Sometimes just with a smile on the street to a passing stranger can make a difference we could never imagine."

The most powerful help you are able to provide is by **setting an excellent example.** Let another observe you living well. He or she may not emulate you, but, unless the other is your child, you may have no greater power to affect an other person's decisions than that. You cannot be responsible for what is beyond your control.

Furthermore, it's not as if there are an infinite number of basic approaches to life. The number is actually small. For example, in the first book of his <u>Nicomachean Ethics</u>, Aristotle claims there are only three.

Shunryu Suzuki: "In the beginner's mind there are many possibilities, but in the expert's there are few."

There may only be one.

However, even if there is only one and you know it by direct experience, it may be impossible to communicate it to someone else. Nevertheless, there's a more effective way than trying to impose your conception of what is good on someone else.

It's to listen deeply in order to discover what he or she thinks would be best. If you think it would be a step in a good direction, perhaps you may be able to help that other person to take that step. [See the relevant blog posts in the "moral well-being" category of my blog if you want more tactics about this.]

The basic idea is to help others to evolve to the next level (and there's always another level). By way of contrast, it's not to attempt the impossible by somehow controlling the decisions of others.

Keep in mind when you meet someone new that most people's lives are disorganized. Though they may look good and smell good, their own priorities may be thoroughly muddled. They understand this about themselves, and they don't feel good about it. They may be stuck trying to prevent others from understanding them as they really are.

Exercise 17

Imagine from now on that all the people you encounter are wearing a sign around their necks that's visible only to you. The sign reads, "Help me feel better about my life." Practice finding out what would make them feel better and, if it's something you think would be good for them, ask yourself how you might help that person get it and follow through.

Goethe: "Treat people as if they were what they ought to be and to help them become what they are capable of being." Benjamin Disraeli: "The greatest good you can do for another is not just to share your riches, but to reveal to him his own." Jack Kornfield: "to love and let go can be the same thing."

The key is to forget about yourself. Especially forget even wondering whether or not you'll ever get anything in return.

For example, suppose that you find yourself chatting at a mixer with a fellow you've never met before. Since he could use your help and yet you don't know how you might help, you'll have to ask. How?

A standard way that usually works well is using FORM. Ask about his Family, Occupation, Recreation, and Motivation (or money). Use ordinary, nonthreatening questions. Are you married? Do you have any children? What do you do? How did you get into that kind of work? What do you like most about it? What do you like least about it? What do you do for fun? And so on.

Listen to what he is saying. Just by giving this person your full attention you are giving him something valuable. Most people feel ignored and unheard. Consequently, they genuinely appreciate it when someone simply pays attention to them.

Body language and tone of voice are critical. Don't try to fake an interest; instead, be genuinely interested. Be alert for some common ground with him and build on it.

The meta-message is: You are important. You are valuable. You are so significant that I'm giving you my full attention. When someone listens deeply and non-judgmentally to what you have to say, how does that make you feel? The gift of attention is a very precious gift.

William James: "the deepest principle of Human Nature is the craving to be appreciated." Dean Rusk: "One of the best ways to persuade others is with your ears – by listening to them."

Pay great attention whenever he expresses any frustrations, problems, concerns, or challenges. Ask about them. Ask about the consequences that these difficulties are causing.

Then ask which better outcome he would like and how achieving it would be an improvement.

Wonder aloud what his next step might be to achieve that better outcome. "How might you be able to get X?" Do a little brainstorming together.

Perhaps you can suggest a way that he can get the result that he wants that he hasn't considered. Since you don't know this person, ask whether or not he has a skill that might be useful in obtaining X? If so, what is it? If not, how else might he obtain X using someone else's skill?

However, avoid the temptation to come up with instant cures for another's problems. His agenda may be different from yours. If it's a valuable goal, help him fulfill his agenda; let go of your agenda.

Stephen Covey: "The most important ingredient we put into any relationship is not what we say or what we do, but what we are."

Rather than trying to control the conversation by talking a lot, control it by asking questions. Spend at least twice as much time listening as you do talking. Enable him to discuss what's important to him. Keep the focus positive and solution-oriented.

Follow up! Get his contact information. The next day mail him a handwritten note mentioning how much you enjoyed meeting and talking with him. Whenever you come across an article or book review or something similar that might interest him, mail it to him.

Treating strangers this way may be very uncomfortable at first. It may exhaust you. However, if you force yourself to do it, you'll quickly find it less and less uncomfortable. You'll do it less and less self-consciously. Eventually, you'll even begin to enjoy it! After all, it's good to help others help themselves.

Mike Rayburn: "It is impossible to give more than you receive."

What does this have to do with killing cravings?

Attention is limited. Though it's possible to flit back and forth quickly between different objects, it's actually impossible to focus on more than one object at a time. The more you focus on others, the less attention you'll have to focus on your own thoughts. Since cravings are thoughts, the more you focus on helping others help themselves, the more you'll help yourself by diminishing the attention you give to any cravings that may arise.

Even when you notice a distracting thought, it is powerless to disturb you unless you get entangled in it. Instead, just instantly let it go and get back to paying full attention to whatever you are doing in the present moment.

Furthermore, when the quality of your encounters improves, you'll need to get less satisfaction from food.

11: Taking Better Control of Thoughts

Did you ever wonder why you are less happy than your dog?

Your dog doesn't worry about global warming. Your dog never fights with teenage children. Your dog isn't concerned about your mother's cancer. Your dog doesn't care that you gained 5 pounds since Christmas. Your dog doesn't have any money problems. Your dog isn't afraid of dying alone.

Again, let's distinguish physical pain from suffering. At least occasionally, sentient beings like dogs and humans have pains. That's normal.

What, though, about suffering? Even a cursory glance at the world reveals an astonishing fact: <u>it's normal for humans to suffer</u>. Most people are not happy. They are frequently dissatisfied. By way of contrast, it's not normal even for other kinds of mammals to suffer.[57]

Why is that?

I think it's because of literacy. Humans are the only animals to have written language.

There's a pattern here we've encountered before: an advance that is a boon for humankind is apt to cause problems for human individuals. There's no free lunch: what's good for civilization costs many individual humans dearly.

Just as the rise of farming, the rise of ranching, and the mechanization of work have had deleterious physiological effects on almost all humans, so the rise of literacy has dramatically increased the suffering of almost all humans.

Given that writing is the most important tool ever invented for the advance of civilization, how can it also be an important source of suffering? Excellent question.

Please notice initially that we should *expect* it to have a major cost. How could a major advance lack a major cost? Please, let's be realistic.

I remember wondering in college what my mind would have been like if I had never heard rock and roll music. Well, there's no way to know. I've enjoyed listening to rock and roll music for decades at parties and while pumping iron, and I'm glad to have it available. However, I've also no doubt that, because I found it entertaining, it has too often distracted me and distorted my experiences.

The good news is this: **Some people, sages, have learned how to diminish suffering and even eliminate it without giving up literacy or other benefits of civilization.**

Again, there's a pattern here we've encountered before. It's possible for individuals to learn how to compensate fully for the price paid for advances to civilization. Because many thinkers have thought that it was impossible, this really is good news.

On the other hand, it's also old news. Though practiced too little, the means to accomplish it have been around for thousands of years. If they hadn't been developed, I certainly wouldn't have been able to invent them. All I've done is to discover them and share them with you.

Let's admit a brute fact: **you suffer a lot.** You are not often genuinely happy. You are frequently dissatisfied.

If you happen to have it, please let go of the thought that there must be something inherently wrong with you. **There's nothing inherently wrong with you.** You are normal, but normal isn't good.

Gotama: "no one who is born is free from aging and death. . . aging and death are rolling in on you. . . didn't you ever see a woman or a man, eighty, ninety, or a hundred years old, frail, bent like a roof bracket, crooked, leaning on a stick, shakily going along, ailing, youth and vigor gone, with broken teeth, with gray and scanty hair or bald, wrinkled, with blotched limbs? . . . didn't you ever see a woman or a man who was sick and in pain, seriously ill, lying in his own filth, having to be lifted up by some and put to bed by others? . . . didn't you ever see a woman or a man one, two, or three days dead, the corpse swollen, discolored, and festering?" Steven C. Hayes, Ph.D., Kirk D. Strosahl, Ph.D., and Kelly G. Wilson, Ph.D.: "The single most remarkable fact of human existence is how hard it is for human beings to be happy . . . Suffering is a basic characteristic of human life. . . Humans as a species are suffering creatures."

If there were no cure for suffering, it would be morbid to dwell on the fact that suffering is normal for human beings. Even if we are lucky enough not to die young, we not only have to endure aging, illness, and death, but we suffer because of our awareness of them. Unlike other animals, we understand our fate.

What happens to us is important to us, which is why it's humiliating to think that we are so powerless over our own destinies. Often we can't even shake powerful emotions like fear, anger, loneliness, and grief.

Because suffering is optional, pointing out the fact of suffering is not morbid. In fact, since it stimulates serious thinking about living wisely or well, it's extremely important.

How can suffering be optional? Given the fact of ubiquitous human suffering, how is living wisely or well possible?

The general answer is that we learned how to suffer and it's possible to learn how to let go of (surpass, quarantine) what we've learned.

We became masters of suffering when we mastered literacy. Literacy enables us to live cut off from direct experience of the natural world. It enables us to live in our thoughts (minds, heads). Suffering (dissatisfaction, discontent, misery, unhappiness) is caused by the separation between our thoughts and reality.

Since we have the option of letting go of our thoughts and thereby ending the separation between them and our direct experience of the world, we have the option of reducing or eliminating suffering.

So to free yourself from the prison of your thoughts is to cure suffering. The more you let them go, the less you'll suffer.

This is not to throw out either language or instrumental reason. Good thinking is necessary for problem solving, and we certainly have plenty of problems to solve. It's getting stuck *incessantly thinking and evaluating*, living in our thoughts, that creates suffering. To end it, all that is necessary is to stop creating it.

Gotama said that in many different ways. He said, for example, ". . .the world turns around these eight worldly conditions. What eight? Gain and loss, fame and disrepute, praise and blame, pleasure and pain. . . an instructed noble disciple . . . understands these things as they really are, and they do not engross his mind. . . Having thus given up likes and dislikes, he will be freed from birth, aging, and death, from sorrow, lamentation, pain, dejection, and despair; he will be freed from suffering."[58]

At least according to him, then, the key is giving up likes and dislikes, "I like this" and "I don't like that." Such evaluations are nothing but thoughts. Furthermore, notice that they are egocentric, self-centered, thoughts. All suffering comes from egocentric thoughts and evaluations.

If so, to eliminate suffering, let go of all egocentric thoughts and evaluations. It's that simple.

If you have never before encountered these ideas, please avoid any tendency you may have to blame yourself (or your parents or teachers). You are not *intentionally* creating suffering for yourself and for those you love. It's not as if life came with an instruction manual on how to live wisely or well that you have ignored. It's just that, so far, you (and your parents and teachers) have not figured out how to practice well in order to live well. This occurred because you have learned from literate humans how to live with minimal contact with what is not human.

For nearly all of the time humans have walked the earth, our ancestors lived in intimate relation to the larger, more-than-human world. It's not an accident that they were not literate. It's only relatively recently, in the era of literacy, in the last 2500 years, that we have concluded that only humans can speak. The natural result has been that we pay almost exclusive attention to, listen to, only other humans and human technology. We have become separated from the larger-than-human with which we have been in relationship from the beginning. It is this separation that has created suffering.

If you are interested in understanding more about this diagnosis, I heartily recommend David Abram's The Spell of the Sensuous.

The oral cultures of our successful ancestors did not enable people to live in the inner world of western psychological experience. Until the development of literacy, our ancestors could not and did not live in their own thoughts. The inner/outer distinction is not a natural distinction. Instead of our modern crown of thorns, our nearly total separation between the human and the other-than-human, our ancestors lived in an intimate relationship with the other-than-human. Yes, for them other humans could speak, but so could wolves, lakes, winds, and mountains. Instead of thinking of the other-than-human as inferior, mechanical, deterministic, or dead as we do, our preliterate ancestors took it to be alive and related to it with awe, wonder, and reverence. They presupposed that the earthly biosphere is where *both* the living and the dead lived. Their animistic perspective was reciprocal and balanced.

By way of contrast, the larger-than-human world does not speak to us literate humans. We have become nearly oblivious to it. We don't listen to it anymore. Instead of being deeply intertwined, our lives and the life of the other-than-human have become largely disconnected.

We have forgotten that our objective science is rooted in the same subjective, everyday world we engage in with our unaided senses. We ignore the fact that our theories are ultimately grounded in the continually shifting, immediate sensory flux.

Some philosophers have noticed this. For example, "Perception, in Merleau-Ponty's work, is . . . this reciprocity, the ongoing interchange between my body and the entities that surround it. It is a sort of silent conversation that I carry on with things, a continuous dialogue that unfolds far below my verbal awareness – and often, even, *independent* of my verbal awareness . . . Whenever I quiet the persistent chatter of words within my head, I find this silent or wordless dance always already going on."[59]

To quiet the persistent chatter of words within your head, just let go of them and focus instead on what is actually going on in the present moment. When thoughts return, as they will, just repeat that process.

It's impossible to unlearn literacy. Fortunately, that's not required.

What is possible is to pay attention to what is actually happening in the present moment. This is the essence of all the meditative and mystical practices that have ever been developed.

Here, finally, is **the ultimate cure for cravings.** If you follow the first 4 steps of The Killing Cravings Method, you will either eliminate or nearly eliminate all cravings that have physical causes from arising.

What, though, about eliminating cravings that have psychological causes? Those causes come from suffering, which comes from separation.

If you will **regularly practice some standard bodily practice (such as zazen meditation)** or other until you get good at it, you will develop the skill to deal with cravings that have psychological causes. If you are temporarily suffering acutely, this will not be possible until you get back to suffering normally; so, for you, it will be a two-step process.

Since cravings come from either physical or psychological causes and you now understand, in principle, how to deal with both kinds, you now understand how to free yourself from cravings.

Understanding how to do it in principle and doing it are not the same.

Cravings are unwanted thoughts. To use a body practice such as meditation is to train yourself how to free yourself from bondage from all thoughts.

What would that freedom be like? Trying to imagine it is a bit like a fish's trying to imagine living outside the water. Even if you could imagine it, it would be just another thought.

Mastering some body practice or other is the final step of The Killing Cravings Method. It is required for killing all remaining cravings.

So, using meditation as an example, how should you practice?

There's no one way that works best for everyone. There are many different ways that work.

It's a bit like this: think of a mountain that has many paths to its summit. The paths are different, but they all lead to the same place. Some people prefer one path, while others prefer different paths. It really doesn't matter which path is selected; what matters is following a path to its end.

Assuming that you do not already have a daily meditation practice, what should you do?

I don't know what you should do. I've never claimed to know that. I've argued that nobody has knowledge of right and wrong. The best I am able to offer you is my considered opinion.

What I recommend that you do is to begin by incorporating into your daily life the rituals from the first 5 steps of The Killing Cravings Method in the next 5 (or 10) months.

Why?

Again, it's difficult or impossible to meditate well if your brain is not healthy (and it's difficult to have a brain that is healthy if your body isn't healthy). By eating, exercising, and resting well and by improving your interpersonal environment, you will be well set up to begin an effective meditation practice.

Then, if you are not already meditating daily, pick a meditative practice. There's no way to tell in advance which practice will work best for you.

I suggest zazen meditation. That's not just because it happens to be my own practice. It's the simplest and, so, the easiest to learn. It requires little or no equipment, and you can begin immediately to "sit" at home.

[Elsewhere, I have provided detailed instructions on how to begin doing zazen meditation correctly.[60]]

Jack Kornfield: "Spiritual transformation is a profound process that doesn't happen by accident. We need a repeated discipline, a genuine training . . . we need to commit ourselves in a systematic way." Saki Santorelli: "Meditation practice requires a disciplined, sustained effort. Yet at heart, mindfulness meditation is about care, about a willingness to come up close to our discomfort and pain without judgment, striving, manipulation, or pretense. This gentle, open, nonjudgmental approach is itself both relentless and merciful . . ."

Here are the initial guidelines to show you how simple it is.

Decide how long you are going to practice—perhaps 2 or 5 or 10 minutes. Set a kitchen timer for that length of time plus enough time to enable you to get seated. Place it far enough away so that you are unable to hear it ticking and yet close enough so that you will be able to hear it when it goes off.

It's best to have a quiet room in which you can sit on the floor facing a blank wall. If you don't have a meditation mat, simply fold a blanket into about a 30" square. If you don't have a meditation cushion or bench, find something such as a rolled up, folded over piece of carpet to sit on so that your butt is higher than your knees.

If you don't want to use a cross-legged posture, just kneel on the edge of the mat facing the wall about an arm's length from the wall. Sit back on the bench or on the meditation cushion held sideways between your ankles or on the carpet held between your ankles.

What's critical is correct alignment of the spine. To ensure that, always keep both knees lower than your hips.

To ensure an initially satisfactory posture, keep your back erect with your belly pushed forward. Keep your shoulders back with your arms relaxed. Let your hands rest on your lap or on a soft pillow on your lap; with palms facing up, put your left hand on top of your right hand (unless you are left-handed in which case you may reverse them) with the tips of your thumbs lightly touching.

Tuck your chin in so that you feel a slight tension in the back of your neck. Keep your neck straight. It helps to imagine two cords, one from the top back of your head and the other from the front center of your chest, supportin   g you from the ceiling.

Lower your gaze to a spot on the wall a foot or so from the floor. Let your eyes go unfocused. Take a deep chest breath or two and, while keeping your back upright and erect, relax everything else. This will minimize muscular tension while keeping you alert.

Eliminate all voluntary movement for the duration of your practice session; in other words, sit perfectly still.

You should now be in a stable position grounded on three points (your two knees and your buttocks) ready to begin. Breathe naturally with your belly. So what should you do?

Simply count your inhalations and exhalations. As you inhale naturally, think *one* silently to yourself; as you exhale naturally, think *two*. As you inhale again, think *three*; as you exhale again, think *four*. Continue in that way until you hit ten and repeat.

If you get lost in thought and forget where you are, just begin again with *one* at the next inhalation.

That's all there is to it.

The key is very simple: <u>whenever you notice that you are lost in thought, instantly bring your focus back to the counting.</u>

When you are able to do that practice for about 15 or 20 minutes without getting lost in thought, you may go on to the next practice, which is simply counting exhalations. By the time you are able to do the second practice for 15 or 20 minutes without getting lost in thought, you will have had plenty of weeks to find additional instruction.

Since they are just thoughts, drop all your expectations.

Charlotte Joko Beck: "Most of us (myself included at times) are like children: we want something or somebody to give us what a small child wants from its parents.

We want to be given peace, attention, comfort, understanding. If our life doesn't give us this, we think, 'A few years of Zen practice will do this for me.' No, they won't. That's not what practice is about. Practice is about opening ourselves so that this little 'I' that wants and wants and wants and wants and wants – that wants the whole world to be its parents, really – grows up."

What you are doing during meditation is actually practicing freedom from your thoughts. Don't try to stop thoughts from arising. If your brain is working, thoughts will arise. When, however, you notice that a thought has arisen, just let it go and get back to your counting.

In this way, you will be practicing being centered in the present moment without getting lost in your thoughts. This is how to practice getting out of your thoughts and into your life.

The practice, then, is very simple. It is not, however, easy to master. Why? Your thoughts don't want to be ignored; your mind doesn't want to be disciplined. Just persist in your daily practice and, once you are doing it for half an hour or more daily, subtle changes will occur that will reflect your increasing peacefulness.

This is particularly true with respect to emotions. Again, there's a self-centered evaluation at the heart of every emotion. The more you focus on it, the more you strengthen the emotion. The less you focus on it, the more you weaken the emotion. Dropping those thoughts is breaking free from emotional bondage.

Instead of riding the emotional roller coaster up and down incessantly like most people, master meditators have freed themselves from that disturbing rising and falling. If you would dearly love to enjoy greater emotional tranquility, start meditating immediately.

Shunryu Suzuki: "Unless you know how to practice zazen, no one can help you. . . Without this experience, this practice, it is impossible to attain absolute freedom."

You'll find resources in the Selected Bibliography that will enable you to learn more about how to meditate or do other body practices. If it is zazen meditation that interests you, I've listed only what I know to be excellent resources. If another kind of meditation or body practice interests you, you're on your own to research it, although, if another kind does interest you already, you probably already have either access to a teacher or to helpful resources.

Avoid the trap of reading a lot about meditation. You've already read enough in this chapter to enable you to begin. The point is to meditate, not just to learn about meditating.

If reading helps you to sit, read. If it doesn't, don't.

Exercise 18

Select one kind of meditation. Learn how to do it correctly. Begin doing it daily, doing a little more each day until you are meditating for at least 20 consecutive minutes daily. 30 consecutive minutes daily would be even better.

David Chadwick: "It's been said, in Zen practice, that your first enlightenment experience is when you decide to practice. It's the first turning."

The best time for most people to meditate is soon after arising in the morning before eating breakfast. Make it part of your morning ritual. You will refresh your mind by emptying it of thoughts and that will set you up for a more enjoyable morning. Doing it early every day will also help you make it a habit. Furthermore, your environment is likely to be more quite at that time.

From now on, if you are following all 6 steps of The Killing Cravings Method, you may be assured that, if a craving arises, it has cause that you understand how to dissolve. Knowing that, and understanding that it is only a thought, just do what you do during meditation: as soon as you notice it, let it go and continue doing whatever you are supposed to be doing.

The first 4 steps will minimize the occurrence of food cravings. Since it seems to be that the default subject for our thinking is encounters, the 5th step will endlessly provide you with ways to improve your encounters by focusing on others, which will provide satisfactions other than food.

Even so, you may occasionally be inflicted by a craving, and that's when to treat it for what it is, namely, just another distracting thought similar to one that arises during meditation. This explains how the 6 steps work together to enable you to eliminate cravings. The 6th step provides critical practice in letting thoughts go.

Sages, who are always master meditators, never suffer from cravings. It's not that they never have cravings, it's that they let them go as soon as they notice them rather than getting entangled in them.

If you have read this book, you now understand how it is possible to end food cravings. In fact, you now understand how it is possible to end all cravings.

Now that you understand what to do, do it. Why not teach yourself how to live in freedom from cravings for the rest of your life? Instead of struggling with cravings, put your attention into your Project and go enjoy a great life.

Ed Courtney: "When it becomes more difficult to suffer than to change, you'll change." Albert Camus: "I shall tell you a great secret my friend. Do not wait for the last judgment, it takes place every day."

12: The Program in Action

If you have done the 18 recommended exercises, you have everything required to translate The Killing Cravings Method into your personalized plan for successfully killing cravings.

Gather your written exercises together and organize them.

Take a blank sheet of paper. Start with 7 columns, one for each day of the week. Divide each column in thirds for mornings, afternoons, and evenings.

Starting with the contents of your morning ritual and your nutritional plan, write in your daily rituals. When will you meditate daily? When will you do at least 20 minutes of serious reading daily? When will you eat?

Add in your twice weekly strength training workouts.

Add in your twice (or thrice) weekly fitness training.

(Are you going to do any additional mild fitness workouts? If so, add them in.)

How many times weekly are you going to help someone new? In the beginning, make that a deliberate goal just twice weekly. It's excellent practice for getting out of your own thoughts and it might even help others. Don't be too surprised if you find yourself doing it more frequently.

Once you've written out your detailed plan, you're done planning. Now go do it.

Tommy Kono: "The day you start to make excuses is the day you will quit making progress." Samuel Johnson: "The fountain of content must spring up in the mind, and he who hath so little knowledge of human nature as to seek happiness by changing anything but his own disposition, will waste his life in fruitless efforts and multiply the grief he proposes to remove."[61]

Thank you for reading this book. May all your dissatisfactions be mild and fleeting, and may all your joys be as profound as they are enduring.

Abbreviations

"BMI" =df. "body mass index"
"DOMS" =df. "delayed onset muscle soreness"
"GXP" =df. "graded exercise protocol"
"NLP" =df. "neuro-linguistic programming"
"OMS" =df. "onset muscle soreness"
"RICE" =df. "rest, ice, compression, elevation"
"5X" =df. "5 meals daily"
"6X" =df. "6 meals daily"

Notes

1. 28e, Grube translation.
2. 38a,Tredennick translation.
3. 517b, Helmbold translation.
4. To read more about this very important idea, I recommend Herrigel's classic <u>Zen in the Art of Archery</u>, Czikszentmihalyi's <u>Flow</u>, and Gallway's <u>The Inner Game of Tennis</u>.
5. Gotama [The Buddha], <u>In the Buddha's Words</u> (Boston: Wisdom, 2005; Bhikkhu Bodhi, tr.), p. 89.
6. For more on self-esteem, go to: http://www.lasting-weight-loss.com/self-esteem.html
7. There's a helpful one, for example, at www.kolbe.com/
8. For example, if you are interested in understanding how your birth order influenced how you came to be as you are, I suggest Frank J. Sulloway's <u>Born to Rebel</u>. (I was, effectively, a first child and, unlike any of my siblings, wound up with an advanced degree just like my father.) For example, if you are interested in understanding the personality similarities between you and other people, I suggest Paul D. Tieger & Barbara Barron-Tieger's <u>The Art of Speedreading People</u>. (I'm an INTJ.).
9. See my <u>Mastery in 7 Steps</u> (Las Vegas: Ironox, 2007.).
10. Descartes, <u>The Philosophical Works of Descartes</u> (Cambridge: University Press, 1931; Haldane & Ross, eds.), vol. 1, pp. 83 & 84.
11. 1094a, Irwin translation.
12. See Chapter 11. This is an important point emphasized in Zen Buddhism as well as in Acceptance & Commitment Therapy.
13. 263e, Cornford translation.
14. For more on self-esteem and how to improve it, go to: http://www.lasting-weight-loss.com/self-esteem.html

The critical point is that, since you are fully in control of your own evaluations, there's no need to suffer through life with low self-esteem.

15. See my Mastery in 7 Steps, Chapter 7.

16. Three helpful books are: James O. Prochaska, Ph.D., John C. Norcross, Ph.D., and Carlo C. Diclemente, Ph.D., Changing for Good, Steven C. Hayes, Ph.D, with Spencer Smith, Get Out of Your Mind & Into Your Life, and Martin Seligman What You Can Change . . . and What You Can't.

17. I have explained it in, for example, Personal Transformation: 5 Ways to Diminish Failure Almost Instantly.

18. See the works of Panayot Butchvarov for the best defense of this claim, particularly The Concept of Knowledge (Evanston: Northwestern University Press, 1970).

19. I can know, for example, that I *seem* to be seeing a tree over there (because it is a present state), but I cannot *know* that I am seeing a tree over there (because, perhaps, I may only be dreaming that I am seeing a tree over there, which would mean that the perceptual judgment was false or mistaken despite seeming real).

20. I discuss perception more in both The 7 Steps to Mastery and Personal Transformation.

21. Understanding the nature of nondemonstrative evidence is the chief problem in epistemology.

22. I have a blog on well-being at http://dennis-bradford.com/ . I took this example from a blog post. If you'd like to read it, simply go to the "intellectual well-being" section of my blog and look up the post entitled "General Adaptation Syndrome Stages." While you are there, I encourage you to sign up to receive my blog posts. They are free, and I believe that you'll find them valuable and stimulating. Furthermore, feel free to leave comments; since I may respond to your comments, that's one way to receive what I hope you'll consider good feedback without spending any money.

23. I also discuss this more in Chapter 10. I agrue against this notion of a "continuant substratum" in several other books. Philosophers such as Gotama, Nagarjuna, and Hume also advocate a reductionist view of the self. For a short excellent discussion, see Chapter 7 in Jan Wester-hoff's excellent <u>Nagarjuna's Madhyamaka</u>.

24. Type 2 diabetes closely relates to the other epidemics of obesity, cardiovascular disease, and autoimmune disease. (I written about this on my blog.)

25. Glucose is the monosaccharide, which is the simplest kind of sugar, that is the chief source of energy for most cells. When blood glucose levels are too high, you have diabetes.

26. I have more training about The Killing Cravings Method available in additional writings as well as in other formats. If you might be interested, sign up for my blog posts, which will enable me to alert you when they become available. Again, it's at http://dennis-bradford.com/ .

27. If you'd like to read more about this, two good books are McRobert's <u>Build Muscle Lose Fat Look Great</u> and Larry Pepe's <u>The Precontest Bible</u>.

28. Don't confuse your percentage of body fat number with your BMI (Body Mass Index) number.

29. There are plastic calipers easily available that you can quickly learn to use efficiently in order to chart your percentage of body fat at home.

30. You may have heard the myth that consuming a lot of protein is harmful for your kidneys. If your kidneys are healthy, that's false. Dietary protein has no substantial effect on the glomerular filtration rate of healthy kidneys – nor does it cause diabetic nephropathy.

31. An inexpensive paperback is Corinne T. Netzer's <u>The Complete Book of Food Counts</u>. Get the most recent edition. Another good alternative is <u>The Nutribase Complete Book of Food Counts</u>. A more expensive alternative is the most recent edition of Jean A. T.

Pennington, ed., <u>Bowes & Church's Food Values of Portions Commonly Used</u>. There are also free reliable online sources.

32. This is an important point: if you will force yourself really to restrict salt intake, your desires for salty foods will soon diminish significantly and lastingly.

33. For specific guidelines on what kind of equipment you'll need to test yourself and how to use it, see the latest edition of <u>Dr. Berstein's Diabetes Solution</u>.

34. The great advantages that unnatural foods have over natural foods is that they are less expensive and more plentiful. Please don't get stuck on the thought that you cannot afford them. Obstructive thoughts like that are nothing but excuses. To open to possibilities, ask, "HOW can I afford them?" In our economic system, you can increase your income by helping others get what they want. Because treating yourself well physically also reduces your chances of ill health, in the long run it can be less expensive to purchase natural foods than unnatural ones.

35. The Buddha, <u>The Connected Discourses of The Buddha</u> (Boston: Wisdom, 2000; Bhikkhu Bodhi, tr.), p. 176. Similarly, Nagarjuna, arguably the greatest Buddhist author, writes: "Take food as medicine, in the right amount, / Without attachment, without hatefulness: / Don't eat for vanity, for pride or ego's sake, / Eat only for your body sustenance." (Nagarjuna, <u>Nagarguna's Letter to a Friend</u>, p. 104.).

36. Scientists are learning more about this all the time. A very good book on this is Brian Wansink, Ph.D., <u>Mindless Eating</u>.

37. See, for example, Julia Ross, <u>The Diet Cure</u>, p. 184ff.

38. Joan Mathews Larson, Ph.D., <u>Depresson-Free, Naturally</u>, pp. 68-70. Also see Julia Ross, <u>The Mood Cure</u>. If you have trouble with alcohol, see Joan Mathews Larson, Ph.D., <u>Seven Weeks to Sobriety</u>.

39. Physicians look at blood lipids (fats) to indicate risk of vascular disease and coronary events (heart attacks and strokes). Your cholesterol ratio is the ratio of total cholesterol to HDL (high-density lipoprotein). It's a good idea always to keep a copy of your lab reports. They will indicate how to interpret the results. For example, the lowest cholesterol ratio for women would be 2.9 or lower and for men would be 3.8 or lower. (A recent one of mine was 3.3.) They may also look at your fasting triglyceride level.

40. How can you tell whether or not a certain food causes a blood sugar spike? Simply buy an inexpensive meter and test yourself after eating it. The best guide I've seen with respect to how to buy and use a meter is in Richard K. Bernstein, MD, FACE, FACN, FCCWS, Dr. Bernstein's Diabetes Solution (N.Y.: Little, Brown, 2007). Don't worry: these days the pain involved in drawing a drop of your own blood is negligible.

41. Is your drinking water clean? If in doubt, have it tested. If it's unsatisfactory and you contact me, I am willing to help you obtain an excellent home water purification system available at the distributor's discount price. It's still relatively expensive, but over time the water you use will only cost you about one-sixth of what most bottled waters cost. I use it myself. Alternatively, check *Consumer Reports* magazine for ratings. Unfortunately, even if a municipality supplies your water, that's insufficient to ensure it's safe.

42. By way of contrast, fats and "simple" carbohydrates only elicit 3% of a meal's total calories, and "complex" carbohydrates elicit a 20% thermic effect. Remember, though, that even so-called "complex" carbs are broken down to simple sugars.

43. The blog is at: www.dennis-bradford.com/

44. I recommend adopting a general perspective like the one provided by Jared Diamond in his The Third Chimpanzee and Collapse . Since the most deleterious

decision a human can have on the environment is the decision to have (and raise) a child, I myself have never done it and never will. (I had myself sterilized several decades ago.)

45. There are plenty of books listed in the back of this book that are very helpful with respect to eating well.

46. It is possible to combine both kinds of exercise by doing what's known as "circuit training." It may be the best alternative for some people and it's certainly much better than not exercising.

47. For Dr. Winet's latest recommendations, see his "Master Trainer" newsletter.

48. CardioSport, Timex, and Polar seem to make good ones.

49. If you are more serious about fitness, you may want to use the Karvonen method of calculation. You can find it at: http://www.lasting-weight-loss.com/running.html

50. Start by going to http://www.lasting-weight-loss.com/walking-for-weight-loss.html

51. I discuss it at http://www.lasting-weight-loss.com/behavioral-weight-loss-tips.html

52. Compare Andrew Weil, Natural Health, Natural Medicine [rev. ed.], p. 169.

53. I analyze the structure of emotions and explain exactly how to get on top of them in Emotional Eating. The central delusion is the belief in a separate, substantial self that I argue against in Chapter 10.

54. I don't get a kickback for recommending this book. At least in its first edition, even McRobert isn't always correct—as I pointed out to him. He wrote me all that would be well in its next revision.

55. If you are an intermediated or advanced trainee and want to know it, contact me; I'm willing to email you a PDF report that details how to test yourself for the optimum number of repetitions.

56. This is the exact point in the dialectic of western philosophy that thinkers like Hume and Nietzsche

challenged thinkers like Aristotle and Descartes. For example, Descartes based his conceptual system on the cogito ("I think"). He presupposed that there is a self, a thinker, doing the thinking. Nietzsche challenged this assumption: "When I analyze the process that is expressed in the sentence, 'I think,' I find a whole series of daring assertions that would be difficult, perhaps impossible, to prove; for example, that it is *I* who think, that there must necessarily be something that thinks, that thinking is an activity and operation on the part of a being who is thought of as a cause, that there is an 'ego' . . . " (From section 16, Beyond Good and Evil, Walter Kaufmann, tr.). For the spiritual practice based on this point, see Bhagavan Sri Ramana Maharshi's Who Am I?

57. They may, for example, suffer from grief or fear occasionally, but suffering is not their normal state.

58. Gotama, IN THE BUDDHA'S WORDS, pp. 32-3.

59. David Abram, THE SPELL OF THE SENSUOUS (N.Y.: Random House, 1996), pp. 52-3.

60. There are more detailed instructions in both How To Survive Collegte Emotionally and The Meditative Approach to Philosophy. There's also a video on how to still yourself physically at: http://dennis-bradford.com/spiritual-well-being/kneeling-meditation.

61. Permit me a personal request: Although I may not be able to respond personally to what you communicate, I'd very much appreciate it if you'd let me know your results after you've worked this program into your everyday rituals for six or twelve months.

What helped the most? What was the most difficult ritual for you? In practice, did any of the written instructions from this book leave you confused? Were you always confident about what you were supposed to be doing? Did you always have a good idea why you were doing it? Where could you use more detailed instructions?

Your feedback may help me to help others in the future. See the About the Author section below for how to contact me via social media or my blog.

SELECTED BIBLIOGRAPHY

Abram, D. The Spell of the Sensuous.
Audette, R., and Gilchrist, T. Neanderthin. **R**
Ballantyne, S. The Paleo Approach.
Bandler, R. Using Your Brain – For a Change.
Bandler, R. and Grinder, J. Frogs into Princes.
Barrett, D. Waistland.
Begley, S. Train Your Mind Change Your Brain.
Biehl, B. Stop Setting Goals If You Would Rather
    Solve Problems.
Blanton, B. Radical Honesty.
Braly, J., and Hoggan, R.. Dangerous Grains.
Bradford, D. 5 Ways to Diminish Failure Almost
    Instantly.
-----. Emotional Eating.
-----. Getting Things Done.
-----. How to Eat Less – Easily! **R**
-----. How To Survive College Emotionally.
-----. It's Not Just About the Money!
-----. Love and Respect.
-----. Mastery in 7 Steps.
-----. Personal Transformation.
-----. The Three Things the Rest of Us Should Know
    about Zen Training.
-----. Weight Lifting.
Butchvarov, P. The Concept of Knowledge.
-----. Skepticism About The External World.
-----. Skepticism in Ethics.
Brown, M. Stone Soup.
Buckingham, M., and Clifton, D. O., Now, Discover

Your Strengths.
Butler, G., and Hope, T. Managing Your Mind.
Carnegie, D. How to Win Friends & Influence
        People.
Challem, J., Berkson, B., and Smith, M. D.
        Syndrome X.
Chapman, G. The Five Love Languages.
Cialdini, R. B. Influence.
Cialdini, R. B., Goldstein, N. J., and Martin, S. J.
        Yes!
Cohen, A. Are You As Happy As Your Dog?
Cordain, L. The Paleo Diet. **R**
----- with Nell Stephenson and Corrie Cordain. The Paleo
        Diet Cookbook. **R**
Csikszentmihalyi, M. Flow.
Descartes, R. Discourse on Method.
Diamond, J. Collapse.
-----. The Third Chimpanzee.
Dogen. Master Dogen's SHOBOGENZO.
        Nishijima & Cross, trs.
Eades, M. R., and Eades, M. D. Protein Power. **R**
-----. The Protein Power Lifeplan. **R**
Fisher, B.. Rebuilding.
Gallway, W. T. The Inner Game of Tennis.
Garfield, J.L. Empty Words.
Giblin, L. How To Have Confidence and Power In
        Dealing With People.
-----. Skill With People.
Gilbert, D. Stumbling on Happiness.
Goleman, D. Emotional Intelligence.
-----. Social Intelligence.
-----. Vital Lies Simple Truths.
Gotama (The Buddha). Basic Teachings of the
        Buddha. Glenn Wallis, ed.
-----. Early Buddhist Discourses. J. J. Holder, ed.
-----. In the Buddha's Words. Bhikkhu Bodhi, ed.
-----. The Dhammapada. Glenn Wallis, tr.

Gladwell, M. Blink.

Groves, B. Natural Health & Wellness. **R**

Hallowell, E. M. CrazyBusy.

Hanh, T. N. Teachings on Love.

Hayes, S. C., and Smith, S. Get Out of Your Mind & Into Your Life.

Hayes, S. C., Strosahl, K. D., and Wilsom, K. G. Acceptance and Commitment Therapy.

Hedges, B. Read & Grow Rich.

Helmstetter, S. What To Say When You Talk to Yourself.

Herrigel, E. Zen in the Art of Archery.

Hume, D. A Treatise of Human Nature.

Huntington, C.W., and Wangchen, G.N. The Emptiness of Emptiness.

Kapleau, P. The Three Pillars of Zen.

Kenton, L. The X Factor Diet. **R**

Koch, R. The 80/20 Principle.

Kubik, B. D. Dinosaur Training.

Larson, J. M. Depression-Free, Naturally.

-----. Seven Weeks to Sobriety.

Lauren, M., with Clark, J. You Are Your Own Gym.1

Lazarus, R. S., and Lazarus, B. N. Passion & Reason.

Loehr, J., and Schwartz, T. The Power of Full Engagement.

Loori, J. D. Riding the Ox Home.

Maltz, M. Psycho-Cybernetics.

Martin, P. The Zen Path Through Depression.

McRobert, S. Build Muscle Lose Fat Look Great.

Merleau-Ponty, M. Phenomenology of Perception.

Nagarjuna. The Fundamental Wisdom of the Middle Way. (Jay L. Garfield, tr.)

Nomura, C., Waller, J., and Waller, S. Unique Ability.

Norretranders, T. The User Illusion.

Pagan, E. "Become Mr. Right" (DVD set).

Plato. Five Dialogues.
Price, W. A. Nutrition and Physical Degeneration.
Pritchett, P. Hard Optimism.
Prochaska, J O., Norcross, J. C., and Diclemente, C. O., Changing for Good.
Ross, J. The Diet Cure. **R**
-----. The Mood Cure. **R**
Sanfilippo, D. Practical Paleo. **R**
Schwartz, D. J. The Magic of Thinking Big.
Sears, A. P.A.C.E.
Smith, M. D. Going Against the Grain.
Stanford, C. B. The Hunting Apes.
Strossen, R. J. Super Squats.
Sulloway, F. J. Born to Rebel.
Suzuki, S. Zen Mind, Beginner's Mind.
Taylor, J. B. My Stroke of Insight.
Tieger, P. D., and Barron-Tieger, B. The Art of Speedreading People.
Tolle, E. The Power of Now.
Wansink, B. Mindless Eating.
Weil, A. Healthy Aging.
Westerhoff, J. Nagarjuna's Madhyamaka.
Wiley, T.S., with Formby, B. Lights Out.
Wolf, R. The Paleo Solution Diet. **R**

About The Author

I was born 3 July 1946 in Teaneck, New Jersey, U.S.A. I grew up in Toledo, Ohio, where I attended Deveaux elementary school and then the schools in Ottawa Hills from grades 5 through 11. I graduated from Blair Adacemy in 1964. I was a pre-professional philosophy major at Syracuse University and graduated in 1968. After two years as an Army lieutenant with overseas duty in Korea from 1969-1971, I attended graduate school at The University of Iowa where I received an M.A. (1974) and Ph.D. (1977). Panayot Butchvarov was my dissertation director.

I taught humanities and philosophy at SUNY Geneseo from 1977 to 2009. Some of the books I've written are listed near the beginning of this book.. I founded the Iron-ox Works, Inc., publishing company in 2004. I do one-on-one coaching/consulting (usually over the telephone).

I'm a former member of MENSA and the American Philosophical Association. I played hockey for many years in the Rochester Metro Hockey League. I've been a member of the Rochester Zen Center for about twenty years. I live happily in solitude in a cottage on the shore of Conesus Lake, which is the westernmost of the Finger Lakes in upstate New York.

For more about me, visit the About me section at consultingphilosopher.com or my Author Central page at http://www.amazon.com/-/e/B0047EI11A

If you'd like to connect with me on social media, just go to: http://www.linkedin.com/pub/dennis-e-bradford/1a/a2a/524/ You'll also find there how easy it is to contact me should you wish to do so. And/or http://www.facebook.com/dennis.bradford.313 as well as http://www.twitter.com/dennisebradford

I encourage you to visit my blog on wisdom and well-being: http://dennis-bradford.com . Its posts are grouped in terms of six kinds of well-being (in no particular order) on the sidebar, namely, financial, moral (interpersonal), intellectual, physical, emotional, and spiritual. I encourage you to begin with whatever interests you most. Please feel free to leave comments. I happen to think that there's an enormous amount of free, valuable content there.

If you are interested in finding out more about getting my help with your own book, go to: http://ironoxworks.com/.

If you are interested in finding out more about my national media citation service for attracting warm prospect to your business (see my photo on the back cover), go to: http://ironoxworks.com/media-authority-publicity-icons/ and watch the video. (My most related books are How to Become Happily Published and 12 Publicity Mistakes that Keep Marketers Poor.) If you are interested in obtaining a substantial discount, instead of ordering directly yourself, contact me and request "the Killing Cravings discount."

If you are interested in finding out more about my other books, they are available in various places, including: http://www.amazon.com. (Simply select 'Books' or 'Kindle store' and do a search for 'Dennis E Bradford').

If you are interested in finding out more about one-on-one consulting with me, go to: http://consultingphilosopher.com/ [Don't fail to use the very special offer in Chapter 4.]

I've a **favor** to ask: will you please go to amazon.com, look up this book, and leave some feedback? I may not be the only one who benefits from your judgment. Thank you.

Printed in Great Britain
by Amazon.co.uk, Ltd.,
Marston Gate.